Healing Birth Healing Earth

Copyright © 2019 Shirley Ward

All rights reserved. No part of this book may be reproduced in any form or by electronic or mechanical means including information and retrieval systems without permission from the publisher in writing.

Ward, Shirley, 1941 –
Healing Birth Healing Earth:
A journey through pre- and perinatal psychology.

Shirley Ward.
ISBN 10: 188076590X
ISBN 13: 9781880765906

Artwork: Ahonu (ahonu.com)
Manuscript editor: Aingeal Rose (aingealrose.com)
Manuscript designer: Ahonu (ahonu.com)

Warning – Limits of Liability and Disclaimer of Warranty
The author and publisher shall not be liable for your misuse of the material in this book. This book is strictly for informational, educational and entertainment purposes only. The author and/or publisher do not guarantee or warrant that anyone following the techniques, suggestions, tips, ideas, or strategies in this book will become successful at anything. The author and/or publisher shall have neither liability nor responsibility to anyone with respect to any loss or damage howsoever caused, or alleged to be caused, directly or indirectly by the information contained in this book. Always consult a licensed health practitioner for all health issues.

Address all inquiries to:
Shirley Ward
Amethyst Resource For Human Development
Ballybroghan, Killaloe, Co. Clare, V94 EE6N Ireland
+353 61 374 533
shirley@shirleyward.org
https://shirleyward.org

Healing Birth
Healing Earth

Table of Contents

Dedication	v
About Shirley Ward	xiv
Part One: Pre- And Perinatal Psychology	1
Ch 1 From Birth Trauma To Primal Scream	2
Ch 2 Frank Lake, His Life and Work	12
Ch 3 Amethyst Resource for Human Devt	38
Part Two: Pre- & Perinatal Influences	44
Ch 4 Birth Metaphor	45
Ch 5 Birth Trauma in the Adult	52
Ch 6 Birth Trauma in Babies and Children	67
Ch 7 Work At Amethyst	78
Ch 8 Traumatic Intra-Uterine Events	84
Part Three: Some Case Studies	101
Ch 9 Case Studies	102
Ch 10 Pre- And Perinatal Work With Adults	110
Ch 11 Experiential Therapy	119
Ch 12 Experiential Psychotherapy	123
Part Four: Wider Implications	132
Ch 13 Fractals From The Womb	133
Ch 14 Narcissism: A Weapon Of Destruction	149
Ch 15 The Human Chakras	168
Ch 16 Global Fractal Waves - A Reflection	183
Ch 17 The Way Forward	198
Bibliography	213
More To Explore	221

Dedication

How we are prepared for conception; the circumstances surrounding our conception; the state of our parents at our conception; how we are treated in the womb; how we are born—influences our lifelong behaviour, and that conclusively, we live our lives according to the trauma or glory of our birth.

~ Shirley Ward

Dedicated to the memory of my parents both born during the difficult days of World War 1, who gifted me with life during World War 2. Their vision was always hope for a brighter future. I have attempted to continue this vision with insight and positivity in my life and the understanding that to help one person is to help to heal the world. Healing our birth and understanding its impact on our life is a great step forward and gives hope for our human race.

Acknowledgements

Grateful thanks to the generosity of Kevin O'Grady (Ahonu) and his wife Aingeal Rose of Twin Flame Productions, Oregon USA (https://twinflameproductions.us) for taking my book, *Fractals From The Womb* and revising, editing and republishing it in this new updated edition, **Healing Birth Healing Earth**.

To the many clients and Amethyst workshop participants, students and graduates who have courageously relived their journey from Conception to Birth not only to heal the past out of their own present but to help make the world a better place to live—thank you.

To Alison Hunter and Carmel Byrne for their skill and dedication to heal our children's children and their continued patience with me.

For all those who have contributed their memories of Frank Lake and his work and to the late Sylvia Lake, Frank's wife for documentation and knowledge of his early life.

To the Clinical Theology Association, now the Bridge Pastoral Foundation for continuing the legacy of Frank Lake's work and integrating it into the newer therapies of the new millennium.

To my friend and mentor Rosalyn Bruyere for the teaching of energy systems in a compassionate and healing way to help dissipate early trauma.

To Dr. Jean Houston for being an ever constant inspiration and for her personal permission to use her creative work and writings in any way I wished for the greater good in developing Human Potential for the Possible Human.

To the late Dr. David Chamberlain for his constant interest, encouragement and belief in our work since our first meeting at the Association of Pre and Perinatal Psychology Conference in 1991. This organisation continues to lead the way globally in the understanding of birth and its effect upon individual lives.

To Ursula Somerville for her persistence in documenting our conversation about my life and work with Pre- and Perinatal Psychology and its effect upon global and planetary issues; and to the Editorial Board of the Irish Association for Humanistic and Integrative Psychotherapy for the publication of the conversation.

To all the pioneers who have founded and researched the area of Pre and Perinatal Psychology upon which Pre and Perinatal Psychotherapy has its roots. It can take a major place in the healing of our planet and how we treat the planet for the future of our children's children—where healing birth can heal humans and transform their treatment of the earth for future generations.

Personal Experience of the Author

Since its founding in 1982 by Alison Hunter, Amethyst Resource for Human Development in Ireland has pioneered and researched the experiential work of over 2,500 people reliving their journey from conception to birth. I have worked with Alison from the beginning.

Over the last twenty five years or more, there has been a timely renaissance of birth memories and hypotheses of intra-uterine and conception memories. Theoretical studies go back at least eighty years to the time of Otto Ranks work in 1924.

Amethyst has at its foundation the work of Dr. Frank Lake, the British psychiatrist who spent many years of his life exploring the realms of conception, the first, second and third trimesters of life in the womb and the affect of these experiences upon later personality and behaviour. I knew Dr. Frank Lake personally. He was the first British psychiatrist to recognise the importance of trauma at birth and before birth in the development of personality. During my time with Amethyst, I have attempted to prove through experiential work and communication with international colleagues, the truth behind his many hypotheses of life in the womb. Very real events occur in the pre- and perinatal period which relate to dysfunction and deprivation, leading to dysfunctional children and adults.

Our work at Amethyst is mainly Humanistic and Integrative Psychotherapy and includes primal integration, regression therapy, energy healing, visualisation, meditation, bioenergetics, artwork, creative story writing, shamanic journeying, dancing and music. The major work is the healing of wounded adults and children whose problems may lie in this uncharted area of life in the womb.

Play therapy, incorporating birth facilitation for children is also a technique used by Carmel Byrne, Child and Adolescent Psychotherapist working at Amethyst.

The Retrieval of Birth Memories

Since his death in May 1982, Dr. Lake's work is now having a major impact upon the realms of pre- and perinatal psychology world-wide. He believed that the behavioural and emotional reactions of a pregnant mother affect her foetus in many ways, which affect the perception of the Self in adult life. His work is being documented and researched by individuals as more evidence is being produced.

The retrieval of pre- and perinatal memories (from before and around birth) and including as far back as conception, can help us understand how and why we behave as we do in the world. The deep parenting and spiritual parenting of our own self-discovery of those primal times, begins to heal what might have gone amiss in the conception, gestation and birth from our physical parents.

Your conception, gestation and birth may be experienced as wonderful or terrible. Remembering helps the re-creation of your Self. It creates the deep healing of what went wrong and the deepening realisation of what went right.

It is important to remember and experience the positive in order to empower your whole being and to overcome the negative blocks which have hampered the development of your human potential. Many answers are found in these periods of human development; the study of which is still in its own infancy.

Two Views On The Nature Of The Unborn

Firstly, scientific studies of the activities of the unborn and newborn baby are being documented—particularly the unborn—with the use of ultrasound scanning of the foetus in utero. From before birth, ultrasound is revealing the hidden life of the unborn baby. We are learning that babies are a source of knowledge in themselves and can teach us much about this early stage of life. Research is being conducted with groups of babies after birth, studying the effects of alcohol, drugs and nicotine upon the new born if taken by mother during the pregnancy. BBC Radio 4 reported that doctors in Sweden in 1979 had made a small study of 69 cases of amphetamine addiction and pregnancy.

Of these 69 women, 17 stopped taking drugs when they realised they were pregnant. The other 52 continued to take drugs throughout their pregnancy. The psycho-social backgrounds appeared to be of significance. It was found that as well as the effects of drug exposure on the developing foetus, children born to mothers who misused drugs during their pregnancy represent a high risk group for behavioural and developmental problems.

For many years, the common scientific practice has been to approach the earliest period of human development as a period of quiet time in the womb where nothing happens. There is a widespread belief that baby simply grows for nine months inside Mother—cosy, warm, protected and comforted. There is also a belief that life begins at birth and not before. Factually, we now know that nothing could be further from the truth.

Two major contributors documenting some of these results are Dr. David Chamberlain, in his book The Mind of Your Newborn Baby and Dr. Tom Verney in his book, The Secret Life of the Unborn Child.

Dr. Chamberlain states that, *"Women have been growing babies from the beginning of the human race, but never with the vision that is possible today."* If mother laughs or coughs, most foetuses will move and respond. He reports that if mothers are violated or assaulted, babies will learn about violence. If mother is loved, babies will learn about love. In one telling incident, a foetus whose mother received an electric shock whilst she was ironing sat bolt upright and immobile in the womb for two days—long after the mother had recovered.

There are signs that mainstream medicine is also looking more deeply into the prenatal period. Peter Nathanielsz MD, who is the James Law Professor of Physiology at Cornell University, presents the case that a lifetime of poor health—from coronary disease and stroke to obesity and diabetes—can start with poor conditions in the womb.

Nathanielsz acknowledges David Barker, who was Director of the Medical Research Centre at Southampton University, as a pioneer in foetal programming. It was Barker's original epidemiological study in the 1980's that found the likelihood of dying of heart disease to be 50% greater in men whose birth weight was less than 5.5 pounds, compared with men who were 9.5 lb babies.

Nathanielsz believes that what we experience in the womb marks us forever. He suggested that somewhere in the womb lie the origins of the diseases from which most of us will die. It is now being hypothesised that what happens in the womb may lead to a whole range of conditions previously associated with getting old. Medical science is now proving that bad memory, heart disease and diabetes can be traced back to the intra-uterine period.

By exploring life in the womb, medical science may be discovering a new model of chronic disease. A major finding is that mum's and dad's need to be encouraged to take better care of themselves and their unborn babies by avoiding nicotine, alcohol and other drugs.

Rediscovering Womb Memories

These scientific hypotheses are not new to therapists working with womb memories. They work with birth and womb experiences relived by adults, children and babies in regression therapies (or other body therapies and hypnosis) that go back to conception and before.

My attention was drawn to the study of intra-uterine trauma and birth trauma in the 1970's. Whilst undergoing counseling training at Leicester University, I came across Frank Lake's work in Nottingham at the Clinical Theology Association (now The Bridge Foundation).

With the help of his work, both theoretically and experientially, and discussing this all with him, I have found many answers to my own problems, for I had been conceived and born while my parents were living through the difficult wartime years in England. Some studies have explored the difficulties wartime babies have experienced.

A Glorious Or Awful Conception?

The most amazing concept arising from my clinical work has been the profound effect of the circumstances surrounding their own conception. When reliving their journey from conception to birth, the knowledge that the state of their parents—physically, emotionally, psychologically and spiritually—plus the environment at their conception, was vital to their well-being as a baby, child and adult.

Our conception may have been glorious or awful. Perhaps we have spent the rest of our lives trying to heal the awfulness of conception without consciously knowing where the feeling comes from. If conception has been glorious and loving, maybe we have become the type of people who love the planet, who take life in their stride and are able to relate in loving and caring ways. Perhaps this is the bliss that many of us were denied.

The whole fractal or rhythmic patterns of our conception may permeate the whole of our life, but we are not aware where the patterns come from and how far back they may go.

In my experience, clients often, in altered states of awareness and consciousness, have told me in no uncertain terms and with great clarity what was wrong at their own conception. They have told me they were not wanted, or that they were really loved. They knew whether Mother was sleeping and at peace, or being hassled, or even assaulted. They knew if and when an abortion attempt was made on their lives but was unsuccessful. They knew when father was loving and caring and attentive or busy, uninterested or missing.

They have struggled as adults to overcome difficulties of autism, personality problems and dreadful intra-uterine events which caused the lack of bonding and connection they so desperately needed as babies and developing children. They have told me when drugs or anaesthesia was being administered. This often reverberated in their later life when being *out cold* helped them to avoid painful situations.

From Conception To Birth

My clients have shared with me the extraordinary story of what it was like for them in utero. It seems that their whole journey from conception to birth has been remembered with remarkable accuracy. The pattern of this first journey had been repeated in their young and adult lives.

They were somehow aware of their parents' emotional state at their conception. Some even describe where they were conceived—whether it was a romp in the fields or in a bedroom with red and white curtains!

If we learn from prenatal times that the womb world is warm, open and a positive experience, then this will predispose our attitude to life as being the same after birth. If our womb experience has been one of fear and anxiety, then surely this will be the blueprint from which we live our lives.

Fact Or Fiction?

It seems that babies in utero are screaming out from their wombs to be understood. Wounded individuals in their young and adult lives have striven to find healing midst their hurts. They have tried to make sense of their senseless pain and have tried to find joy in their joyless world. We should begin to take them seriously to help eradicate unnecessary pain and disabling events for future generations.

They have spoken to me of terror, fear, abuse and anger. They have spoken softly to me of peace, joy, love and caring, depending on the womb and family they were born into. They have recalled cold rooms, bright lights immediately affecting their eyes, rough hands, pressure of forceps, good nursing, gentleness and the pain of injections.

They mentioned being suspended by their feet and being smacked and the hasty cutting of the cord. They still feel and live the sense of separation, abandonment and isolation in incubators and hospital wards. They have told me their stories of their birth journey and life journey. If we choose, we can discover the links and similarities between them and heal what we can to live a better quality of life.

Resonance From The Womb

There is a resonance, bodily or emotional response–or sympathetic vibration or energy–between the state of the parents before and at the conception of their child. From this point they can affect the future adult life of their child. This resonance may be found between scientific womb discoveries and future parents understanding what is happening to their baby in utero. There is a resonance between better birthing practices as advocated by Judith Crowe and others such as the

Doulas, water birthers and home birthers to give opportunities for a brighter vision of the future of humanity on the planet.

There is a resonance between the process of individual therapy at the primal level and the future healing of humanity. Conscious regression enables us to reclaim the energy to become much more enlightened and wiser human beings as we traverse into the new millennium. Never before have we been asked to become stronger physically, emotionally and spiritually, as the world becomes insecure in so many ways for all peoples. The fears and anxieties of us all are present as we travel from birth to death and ponder on the possibility of death taking us into new life, or nothing. There is no shortage worldwide of research into the hidden life of the unborn baby (from babies in utero to adults) reliving their journey and looking for empowerment and understanding. They are looking for the deepening of the good things and the healing of the less-than-good things.

Our Responsibility

Whatever our status in life, all human beings are responsible for the evolution and development of the future. The only sin is ignorance and we all have a responsibility to change this. Belief in birth memories and before, is a difficult concept to grasp and a possible one that many sceptics would prefer to deny. The idea of this work is not to frighten future parents, but to impart vital information of these uncharted territories. It is a concept of the utmost importance, which we must understand and believe, for the future of our children's children. The responsibility lies with us all.

SHIRLEY WARD
Ireland 30th June 2019

About Shirley

Shirley Ward lives, works and plays in Killaloe, County Clare, Ireland. Born in Peterborough, England, she was educated at Bedford College of Physical Education, pursuing the life of a professional sportswoman until a knee injury prevented her from continuing.

Educated also at Leicester and Nottingham Universities where she became involved in 1976 with the work of Dr Frank Lake, the first British psychiatrist researching foetal consciousness and life in the womb. Discovering that her own knee injury and negative life patterns related to her own very difficult birth she has for over 40 years, continued researching life in the womb and its effect upon adult personality and behaviour, helping others find answers to negative behaviour.

She moved to Ireland in 1986 working as an educator, healer, and psychotherapist specialising in the pre and perinatal field. Her work is recognized in *'Who's Who in Catholic Life'* and acknowledged also in the *International Biographies Directory* produced by Cambridge University.

She is continuing to expand her knowledge and work alongside the idea that in time healing birth will heal the earth. Removing negatives from the early conditioning and trauma in the pre and perinatal period will assist humans in treating our planet with compassion.

CONCEPTION

The harmonious silence was complete
Within the depths of the oceanic bliss of eternity.
Sleeping, and yet not sleeping.
Knowing and yet not knowing.
Conscious and yet not conscious.
Alive, and yet not alive.
Resting within the sanctity of universal love
Resting and waiting; alone and yet not alone.

The rhythmic patterns of the universe,
The fractal rhythm of auric colours
Permeating eternal sleep.
Light cascading upon light,
Radiating stars beaming their presence
From Eternity.
Rays upon rays.
Multi-fractional rainbows streaming forth.

Strength upon strength, an energy connection
Pulling and pushing, love abounding.

A cracking, resounding, resonating gravitational pull
And a falling from heaven, from infinity.
Tumbling, floating, spinning, spiralling, whirling
Faster, slower, faster
Descending from a great height
Light penetrating light
Resisting, succumbing, allowing
Restraining, choosing, selecting
And with an explosion
Crashing through the
Cosmos Into Conception.
A spiritual being into a physical body.

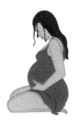

Ursula Sommerville In Conversation With Shirley Ward

Introduction: This conversation concerns my life and the healing influence of pre and perinatal psychology, or healing birth, upon it, and upon the lives of others.

Early negative imprints may be brought into consciousness, be transformed and give a better quality of life. Positive traits may also be recognised and truly transform what may have been unrecognised gifts, that have been dormant since birth in all of us; and this is real human potential.

Understanding the impact of life before birth, both positive and negative, will transform our behaviour to heal and save the planet—or we will continue to destroy and plunder our common home through our own ignorance, disrespect and greed, and negative characteristics we think cannot be changed.

This conversation was published in *Inside Out*, The Irish Journal for Humanistic and Integrative Psychotherapy. No 87. Spring 2019. Published by The Irish Association for Humanistic and Integrative Psychotherapy. 40 Northumberland Avenue, Dun Laoghaire, Co Dublin.

Ursula: *Shirley Ward is, among many things, a founder member and Honorary member of IAHIP and a pioneer of pre- and perinatal psychotherapy. She granted me the great privilege of a conversation which I look forward to bringing to our members here.*

Ursula: I want to thank you for agreeing to have this conversation Shirley and sharing with our members what life can be like following 'retirement'. But before we talk about that, I would love to know what it was that brought you into psychotherapy in the first place?

Shirley: My own problems!

Ursula: Ah, like a lot of us!

Shirley: Some of these problems were on a conscious level but in retrospect many were on an unconscious level and I needed the depth work for healing.

Ursula: So, what was your original training?

Shirley: I trained as a teacher and was also a professional sportswoman, but due to a knee injury had to retire at 24. I changed from physical gymnastics to spiritual gymnastics because my search for personal spirituality was ever present. The knee injury turned out to be associated with a difficult birth. The physical and mental pressure of professional sports reiterated the points of the original stress which had weakened the knee joint.

In the 1970s, I was head of religious education in charge of community development in a large Catholic comprehensive school. Being sensitive to the needs of children with problems in school, I trained as a school counsellor at Leicester University for two years. During this course my own personal problems begin to rise. I asked the tutors if they knew of a Christian therapist and they suggested Dr. Frank Lake and the Clinical Theology Association in Nottingham. And so it all began. I went in the deep end head first. A great birth script!

Ursula: Yes, that's twice you have referred to birth in your responses and I want to talk about your work in pre- and perinatal psychotherapy and the influence that Dr. Lake had on you, but first tell me about your early life.

Shirley: I was conceived, born and lived under the spiritual energy of the great cathedral church of St. Peter and St. Paul in Peterborough. It had been a medieval Benedictine community. I always loved the sacred space it created for me. I walked through many energetic dimensions of life and death in this environment. I have never questioned the existence of a force higher than myself because I experienced it daily in those formative years and always knew of its existence. By the age of four, I had the words refectory, lavabo and cloisters in my vocabulary. I was marinated in energy that deep within filled me with hope and optimism. So much of my belief that environment is above and beyond nature stems from this early period of my life. Environment is the pinnacle upon which all human behaviour, character, health and responses are formed. In England I found peace with the Grail Society and now in later life I find solace at Glenstal Abbey when I am able to go.

Ursula: I don't want to miss the opportunity to hear more about the energetic dimensions of life and death in your environment at that time, but let's come back to that again and for know continue with your early life.

Shirley: from the age of 11 to 22, I helped my mother nurse my sick father who died of multiple sclerosis at the age of 48. The MS was thought to be brought on by the trauma of the Second World War. We were also told medically that Peterborough was an area with a very high ratio of MS due to the removal of minerals in the ground caused by the brickmaking industry after the war. Having to cope with my mother's grief was influential in my decision not to marry as the pain of loss was too great for me at that time. Having no siblings made it more difficult and I struggled through school and college, but my physical abilities got me through with a lot of success on the sports field.

My intelligence and human potential became unblocked the more I let go of the negative patterns in my life. After converting to Catholicism in my 20s, I became a nun at the age of 27 and lasted for four years. I never regret those years. In many ways I continue to learn so much on so many different levels. I was not your usual 'run-of-the-mill' nun. I coached hockey in a red tracksuit with a blue and white veil flying behind me! In 1968 it was the time when nuns were having fashion shows before they went into 'mufti'. In obedience I had to teach classics, knowing very little about the subject so I took classes to see the film *Ben Hur*. I then organised a school cruise to Athens through the Corinth Canal and beyond. We had a great time —but I was verbally flogged by the Mother Superior and Novice Mistress for not asking permission to go. The convent and I went our separate ways two months after we returned from our classic journey —never to be forgotten.

Ursula:[laughing] I'm sorry to laugh Shirley, but it's hard not to at the image of you on the hockey field with a flying veil!

Shirley: You would have laughed even more if you had seen the underwear I had to wear under the novice's long habit. Remember, I was used to wearing shorts, miniskirts, T-shirts and bikinis. Suddenly I had to wear a heavy Aertex vest, the length of which came to between my knees and ankles. It was unbelievable. On one occasion I ran up and down the length of the Novitiate in it and the novices couldn't believe their eyes but still fell about laughing. This was the only way I could accept having to wear it!

Ursula: That's so funny Shirley.

Shirley: On with the serious stuff. Although the emotional problems of parental illness and financial difficulties were overwhelming, nothing has ever prevented me from believing that there is something out there that is beyond our human understanding. I often feel I am on this earth but I am not of it. And I meet so many others who say the same. But I found that I have enormous resilience and determination to discover and pioneer new ways of working to help others to move forward in their lives. This is a major birth script of mine. When I feel stuck —keep moving forward without the pain of the forceps. There are different ways to transform difficult situations.

Ursula: I know your faith is very important to you. However, the aspect of birth script has entered again in our conversation and I think birth script is something you may have learned from working with Dr. Lake and the pre- and perinatal psychotherapy; so can you speak a little about it here?

Shirley: Finding Frank Lake and his work in 1976, and Alison Hunter, one of his pastoral consultants who founded Amethyst in 1982, changed my life. I fell into the pre- and perinatal work. It answered so many questions I thought were unanswerable. It was not only birth scripts that became life scripts but the whole experience from conception to birth I found that formed me as a whole person. I knew that I had to dedicate my life to finding out the truth about womb-time in order to help others understand their own problems. I was lucky to be able to explore the trauma of being a war baby. Saying this, my heart goes out to all babies born in war situations, conflicts and traumatic situations and the effect that this has on personality and mental illnesses. I needed the depth work of pre- and perinatal work to attempt to heal the damage associated with my prenatal growth from conception in December 1940 to my birth in September 1941. The Battle of Britain raged, the bombs were dropping, and fear of annihilation marinated the nation. The terror inflicted on pregnant women and the negativity passed on to babies in the womb is horrific and can have lifelong consequences with mental illness. I know, I have been there —even though I have a deep inner core from my early spiritual experiences. The overwhelming transmarginal stress in trimester three during pregnancy can cause unbelievable mental damage to a baby which is present in many adults for the rest of their lives. So much more research is needed.

Ursula: Yes, and knowing this I have great concern and distress with the amount of war and displacement in the world right now and so many children caught up in it also, children born and those about to be born.

Shirley: It can take years to get the insight as to why we behave as we do. For years I had a real fear of what the next trauma was going to be in my life and I also have been very hampered by sudden lapses of confidence which stopped me in my tracks on projects I wanted to do. Then I saw the light —it was my mother's fear of where the next bomb was going to drop and would she be able to keep me safe. I had to differentiate what were her emotions still affecting me, which I didn't need, and what were mine. I had to remember with compassion that she was born in the First World War and now here she was pregnant in the Second World War. My dream is that more people would've trained to understand pre-and perinatal work. Now I just get on with the job in hand, knowing I am perfectly capable with the potential needed and there actually was an historical place where these feelings originated.

My dream is that more people will train to understand pre- and perinatal work. Consequently, I've spent over 40 years of my life researching foetal consciousness. I have a passion to find out why the human race behaves as it does. It starts in the womb —but few want to know about it. So many mums-to-be are not even aware what smoking and alcohol does to their unborn babies even though it has been medically proven.

Ursula: You have tried to bring this message where you can over your years of work?

Shirley: Yes, I have lectured internationally in USA and Europe, including Russia, France, England and Ireland. I spent months during the 1990s at the United Nations in Vienna where there was enormous interest, often with 28 different nationalities present, and my words being translated into German, the language of the UN in Austria.

But I can't continue without mentioning the wonderful people I have met on my travels and who have influenced my life and teachings. In 1974, I meant Mother Teresa of Calcutta in Birmingham as I ran the Co-Workers for her in Northampton. It was a timeless moment that has stayed with me for life. In 1981, my travels brought me into contact with Rosalyn Bruyere and her wonderful healing work and we have been friends for over thirty years. In 1984, Dr. John Rowan became a Patron of Amethyst. In 1985, after studying for my degree in human relations, my paths crossed with Dr. Violet Oaklander, a wonderful child therapist in California.

In 1986, I give up teaching in England and came to Ireland for two weeks and I'm still here 32 years later. I came over because we had prayed for peace in Ireland daily and then I found I was just coming home. It has been a great privilege to work with Alison Hunter and Carmel Byrne at Amethyst to help adults, children and babies to heal their lives, and to teach students to go out and spread the word and continue the healing.

In 1987, Dr. Jean Houston was invited over to Ireland by the teachers in Dundalk. I met her again in Washington DC in 1991 when I attended the conference run by the Association of pre- and Perinatal Psychology and Health (APPPAH), where I heard from her about the concept of Fractals. It was also here that I met many of the pioneers and founders of pre- and perinatal work, including Dr. Thomas Verney, Dr. William Emerson, and Dr. David Chamberlain, who invited me to become an international adviser for APPPAH and really helped me to feel part of this great community which has continued since then.

Ursula: Not to mention your training in Amethyst and the work that you write about in your book *Fractals From The Womb: A Journey Through pre- and Perinatal Psychotherapy* (2014). I reference this book all the time in my work as a psychotherapist and supervisor. I would like to see more emphasis on it also in current trainings for psychotherapists. You have lived a very full life. Retiring at the age of 70 and being awarded Honorary Membership of IAHIP in 2011. Having served the organisation in multiple ways: founder member, Chair of the Accreditation Committee and Secretary for two five-year stints, Chair and then Secretary of Complaints Committee, Vice Chair of IAHIP in 2003 when when you created a new logo for IAHIP, and 11 years' service on the Editorial Board of *Inside Out*. People know you for your writings in *Inside Out* since 1993. You have also advertised IAHIP globally with your internationally published papers. I think that you were also included in the *European Who's Who in Catholic Life*, and in 2006 and 2011 were selected as one of the best 100 Educators. I hope I haven't left anything out. But, here's the question —what have you been doing since becoming an Honorary Member?

Shirley: Life hasn't stopped. It's almost got busier! I wasn't prepared for life after 70 to be governed by all of my earlier life experiences.

I was always a prolific writer particularly with the pre- and perinatal psychotherapy for *Inside Out* and international journals. I had written other books on masses for teenagers in 1978 and 1983, but *Fractals From The Womb: A Journey Through pre- and Perinatal Psychotherapy* was published in 2014. This is being republished at present by a different publishing firm in the USA, set up by one of our Irish Amethyst students in Oregon.

There is a second book in the pipeline on *Birth, Earth and our Future*. I firmly believe the first nine months of life gives us the foundations of our character and life. The state of parents at conception, the way we are treated in utero and type of births we have influence the way we interact with each other and the planet. This interaction or intercommunication was decide the future of the planet. It is not left to other people —we are all individually responsible for the future of the planet. This in turn leads to Collective Intelligence, Collective Energy, and Collective Interaction for worldwide sensitivity and healing for

xxiii

the planet. At least there is a dream to achieve healing for the care of our common home globally.

Ursula: These are beautiful words to live by: "achieve healing for the care of our common home globally". Thank you for that Shirley.

Shirley: I have also trained as a Minister for Lay Led Liturgies in the Catholic Church in the Killaloe Diocese and have already led communion services, when the priest was abroad. He consecrated the communion hosts at a mass before he left. I love it and I'm passionate to see the lady in charge of their own parishes with the declining number of priests. It's only going back to the early church as in the Acts Of The Apostles.

Dioceses are now training Pastoral Workers as a new vocation to assist priests and then to be ready to take over when there are even fewer priests. I am very excited about this but in a meeting, I asked the Bishop if he would produce a shorter course for the over 70s. Everyone laughed and clapped but the Bishop said I was already trained and to keep on with what I am doing!

Ursula: I can pick up the excitement in you as you talk about this part of your current life. But I'm also hearing that you thought you required further training in this field —what is it that sometimes we don't fully get that we have done enough in our life course and it takes another to tell us what we are capable of doing, in other words, is this also part of our birth script?

Shirley: We are conceived and come into life with enormous potential according to the environment we are marinated in, the negative events on our sacred journey from conception to birth are the problems that need cheering. They fog up our whole life unblock and block our potential. We need the integration of our life story in order to move forward freely and know what we can do. Then we don't need others to tell us what we can do.

Ursula: This seems a good place to ask you to expand on that energetic dimension of life and death in your environment early in your life, is there more you can say here?

Shirley: Remember that my womb and early life experiences were enhanced by death all around, in the country, Europe and the world. We lived opposite a cemetery and the Cathedral was next door. From this environment of sacred and spiritual energy I grew up quite naturally aware of a sixth dimension. The Cathedral had over a thousand years of prayer permeating the stones and I was absorbed by it.

People love solving mysteries. The mystery of life and death we can't solve until we reach that energetic dimension in our lives, but its there for us to tap into. There is much more understanding these days of the chakras and human energy Field with so many complementary medicines being practiced in the country from spiritually active countries. When we receive prayer our energy healing, it may not be used immediately but hangs around for 10 or 20 years or more until we need it. That is the real mystery and is what I tapped into in my early years. It is as natural for me to speak to those who have passed over as it is for me to speak to the living. The church has been speaking to dead people for over 2,000 years so I'm not doing anything that hasn't been done before.

Ursula: Thanks for that Shirley. So can I now bring us more present and enquire what is happening for you now?

Shirley: I was elected Chair of the Ogonnelloe Seniors Club for 2018 in a very thriving, compassionate, caring community. In a year I have also learned how to work with mosaics and stained glass. Now I am drawing animals and learning how to paint with watercolours. As we get older, we need to learn new skills in order to grow new new neural transmitters and the brain to keep ourselves healthy. I am also learning how gentle, spiritual and caring the rural communities of Ireland are, with the quietness and humility it is possibly hard to practice in busy, industrial towns. The land itself is rich which sacred energy.

Ursula: Keeping ourselves healthy is paramount in our work as psychotherapists. Have you experienced or avoided ill health or burnout while working in this field?

Shirley: I haven't avoided it. Illness can really educate us and it can cause our death. In 1992, Allison Hunter and I worked and lectured in Moscow after the Chernobyl disaster. We both came home with radiation poisoning, which in many medical circles is not recognised. I ended up with a serious thyroid problem that eventually affected my heart, which is now under control with medication. But in 2014 when I was 73, an external event of which I had little control, traumatised me and I was hospitalised three or four times and eventually underwent major surgery in 2016. I have to wait for a prognosis, and during those months prepared myself for death. I was one of the lucky ones. After that, I made the decision that I had been given back my life and needed to serve humanity by sharing what my life's work was proving, be it 50 or 100 years ahead of its' time. Hence, another book!

Ursula: I want to go back little on what you were saying about your second book and ask if there's anything you were able to add about how does Collective Intelligence, Collective Energy and Collective Interaction can happen in a world that seems to me to be so divided and, well, broken?

Shirley: Another word of course, is interconnectedness. It is up to individuals and groups to make this happen. I always searched for some of the finest minds to learn from. Jean Houston has been a great mentor for me and she speaks of the rising of our collective intelligence created from the 'world mind', unique she says in its capacity to interact at all levels, and this 'mind' is seeking solutions as an incredible rate. Our recent course is on Quantum Powers, which includes using our power with the energy of the universe and planet earth. The Ocean Rescue project sponsored by Sky is only one of many projects founded by inspirational people. I believe it can happen and Jean Houston encourages us to nurture our imagination and as Einstein did, tap into a deep well of greater possibilities for co-creation with planet earth and the universe. We are the ones truly responsible for the future.

Ursula: The Ocean Rescue project is about everyone making small everyday changes that collectively lead to big changes, this ties in with Yung's thinking that if we can look after that which is in front of us then collectively there will be changes, and here I am thinking of psychotherapy. Do you have any thoughts on psychotherapy and psychotherapists today, since, as you say you first trained in the 70s and became involved in this work?

Shirley: Yes. I don't agree with the way in which all students who train for psychotherapy today have to have a degree. I was fortunate as I studied for a degree in human relations (of all things!) when I was 40. I believe this part of the necessary criteria is barring so many good people from training, who have wonderful life experiences and would make excellent therapists.

We are all so richly unique, I just hope that individuals follow their own dreams and do not worry about being different. We are lucky to have experienced our own therapy, not just to pass our intended courses, and to make a living, but to make the world a better place. The future of planet earth for our children's children is in our hands, as we help those who struggle to find sense in their lives in the therapy room. With a higher energetic understanding of that, as a profession we can help to change the world. However long it takes —but it has to happen.

Ursula: I am thinking of you on the hockey field with your veil flying after you in your red tracksuit, and I also remember working with you on the Editorial Board of *Inside Out* and one thing that always struck me was your sense of humour. In this work of psychotherapy and now with your sense of world healing have you maintained your sense of humour?

Shirley: Yes. I have always had a great sense of humour, if people take the time to hear it. In fact, readers may pick up on it as they read this conversation. Sometimes I am too quick for my own good. It's partly genetic as my mother and grandmother were very funny. Using humour to get through dark and difficult days, my grandmother raised six children during the First World War as my grandfather was a abroad for four years in the war.

My great-grandmother was a Farren and there are connections somewhere to Elizabeth Farren, the Irish Comedienne who was on the London stage in the 1800s for 20 years. I love humour but sometimes I can get myself into trouble with the speed of the humour and I have had to learn to be more sensitive! I am also a Libran so naturally have the ability to balance out both sides of a story. And I just love to listen and read other people's stories. Listening to others makes our own world so much richer.

Ursula: So, you could not have chosen a better profession to work in when you talk of loving listening to other people's stories. I know you live in a beautiful part of Ireland and you've described the community aspect of it earlier. I know also that you have, I think, three cats which are very important to you also.

Shirley: My cats are very precious to me. I have Tonkinese triplets, and they are a Siamese and Burmese mix and would be the temple cats in the Orient. My red boy is Runi Manu. My brown boy is Tomi, named after Tom Brown's schooldays because he was so mischievous as a kitten, and still is. My blue boy is named Stani as the litter was born on St. Stanislaus's day. Oh yes! I have been Chair of the Midland Cat Club of Ireland for 17 years and help Carmel who is the show manager, to run the cat show every February.

Ursula: Before we close our conversation Shirley, what does a day in your life look like?

Shirley: Besides all the things I mentioned, outside in the field we have the local farmers ponies to help keep the grass down. There are two tame male pheasants strutting about. The dawn chorus wakes me often at 4am and during the day there are a great variety of birds around the bird table.

I watch the swallows come and go each year in April and September. I love the peace of being with the animal world.

For those who know us at Amethyst, Allison, now 86, who is also an Honorary Member of IAHIP, has been confined to bed now for nearly three years. Carers come in for five hours a day to her and Carmel is her main carer. So, I try to see Allison or phone her every day. She is not able to sit beside the bed as she has Lymphoedema with legs that do not work due to polio when she was 20.

Ursula: Shirley, I am sorry to hear this about Allison; readers will remember the lovely conversation Allison had which Sarah Kay in this journal back in Autumn 2011. If they have not read it yet it is well worth visiting our website and reading it.

Shirley: Of course Ursula, I agree. This brings me to the reality of today alongside everything else that is going on. I have a home help three times a week, I'm on eight drugs a day. I have on hand a social worker and an occupational therapist who has provided me with a bath seat. I have a good doctor and good friends. I have no family in Ireland. Many in England have passed over —but I talk to them. I have an emergency alarm on the wall that talks to me and tells me when the main power goes off during an electric power cut. When I answer, I am reminded of Shirley Valentine who talked to the wall!!

Sometimes the arthritis is bad and I have a shopping scooter which I take to the shopping centre or go for walks along the Promenade at Lahinch. Ironically it does 4 km/h. I laugh as in my 20s I was an amateur rally driver and speed has been part of my life. When the M1 in England was built, my then boyfriend was a fanatical car mechanic with a 'Baby Austin' with double cylinder heads. The M1 had no speed limits or no speed cops so we raced up and down the motorway at well over 100 mph. This is why I always drive Subaru cars and now have a vintage one which serves me well, with the speed limits in force today!

Ursula: Hmm, rally driver, just as well there are speed limits Shirley, and there seems to be no stopping you in many aspects. I would give you the last word but I want to thank you very much for allowing me to listen to you talk about your fascinating life and I believe, in your sharing, giving others a glimpse into a life after retirement. I like to think of not retiring from something as much as retiring to something and I think you have certainly demonstrated this to us.

Shirley: Thank you Ursula for giving me the opportunity to share my life and work with you. I am always aware that like all of us, the cats, the ponies, the birds of the air and pheasants are survivors, and have been since conception. The ovum and sperm made it, to create each one of us as we are. We made it— and there is still a lot of living, loving and caring to be done.

Life is precious. We are all survivors. May life be good to our readers as they travel under sacred journey of life and thank you for reading my story. You asked me Ursula, in the beginning, what life can be like following retirement. This is it—for me! Older age is like any other age—you learn to adapt!

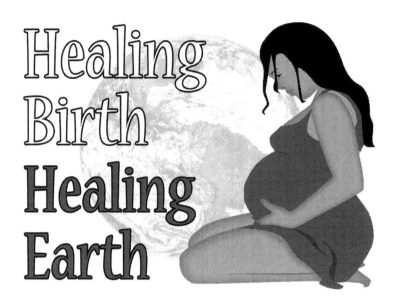

PART ONE

Chapter 1

FROM BIRTH TRAUMA

TO THE PRIMAL SCREAM

Feelings From The Womb

From the beginning of human life, the need for rebirth has appeared in cultural and tribal traditions and rituals throughout the world. We are born onto a planet spinning in a solar system on the rim of a small galaxy, marinated in the energies of a vast universe. The search for the meaning of life—life as individuals, as family, as part of humanity, the urge in the human mind to keep seeking— is constant. We are born only to know one major truth and that is that *we are born to die*. Our most life challenging transitions or transformations are birth and death. It is at the cellular level that both occur. Birth and death are inter-related.

For thousands of years from Egypt to Einstein, the human mind has tried to understand our living universe and the relationship of our human consciousness to the cycle of birth and death. Caldwell implies that there is no birth without death. Birth psychology and death psychology may be taught together. In speaking to mothers on this subject, many of them emphatically say that during the birth process when they were giving birth to their children, it often felt like a dying process for them as well. Birth itself, in birth trauma and before, may also be felt as a death by individuals.

Even from the earliest pioneers of birth work, the search for discovering the unknown, of letting go into unknown dimensions, has and always will be, the fundamental mystery of the search for the understanding of our human situation. This I believe, has been my own underlying passion in searching, exploring and discovering the depths of birth and before, and of being able to help myself and others to move humanity to a new consciousness and realisation of life in the womb and its ultimate consequences on adult life.

Linking in with the work of these early pioneers is a bonding with the development of humanity itself, combined with evolution and the constant search for the mystery of life and death. The development of new insights of our coming into life at conception, nine months in the womb and our birth is bringing forth startling new experiences that impinge upon our entire lives. The early pioneers probably had no idea the part their work would play on this evolution of a new consciousness for humanity.

So much of what we need for understanding ourselves and our future has been hidden in the depths of our first nine months on earth inside our mothers' wombs. Life from conception is truly an adventure, a mystery unfolding the reasons for being who we are, a sacred and spiritual journey for each of us, if we all have the courage to be.

One of the earliest documented accounts of the feeling life of a baby in the womb is in St. Luke's Gospel when Mary visits Elizabeth who was six months into her pregnancy. When Elizabeth greeted Mary, the baby leapt in her womb.

In 1991 a bibliography of pre- and perinatal psychology mentioned a report dated 1867, written by Dr. James Whitehead. He described an unborn child's reaction inside mother's womb when mother was stressfully nursing a two year old very sick child for three weeks. The unborn baby protested against the long stress and discomfort with a violent bout of kicking, lasting about three hours. Michael Irving, editor of the bibliography, states that Dr. Whitehead made an astute observation which preceded the field of birth psychology by over a century; in the mid-19th century it had been noted that mother's emotional state and external circumstances may be felt and responded to by the pre-born in the womb.

The Development Of Various Approaches

One of the major explorations in this field is how to access the memories of birth. The following people and their work all contributed to this phenomenon. It has been a combined contribution over the years of the synthesizing of so many people's exploration and work.

There were experiments in the 1890's in Paris and New York using hypnotic techniques to retrieve birth memories, but as Chamberlain emphasizes in his book, *The Mind of Your Newborn Baby*, there were no verbatim accounts. The idea seemed so preposterous that it received little scientific attention.

Josef Breuer 1842-1925

Breuer can, to some extent, be regarded as the grandfather of psychoanalysis. Breuer sent an account to Freud of a case in which he had looked after the notorious *Anna O* case at the beginning of 1880. It led Freud to the source of the theoretical development of psychoanalysis. Breuer was Freud's best older friend. However, the effects on Breuer of working with *Anna O*, led him to become very frightened of his abreacting (i.e. discharging of emotions) patient, and also his own relationship with his wife. The therapy, called the *Cathartic Method*, consisted of the patient's recall which reproduced forgotten scenes whilst under hypnosis. Freud encouraged Breuer to write about the case, and for the two men to write together a monograph entitled, *Studies on Hysteria*. Their work was poorly received by the medical profession and their friendship ended.

William James 1842-1910

Whether Freud was aware of the work of William James or not, or vice versa, in 1875 James began teaching psychology and set up the first laboratory in America in experiential psychology. His writings include points on *'primary memory'*, in which he suggests that for a state of mind to survive in memory, it must have endured for a certain length of time.

He published, *Principles of Psychology* in 1890. He was aware of the phenomenon of memory, stating that *'memory proper'*, or secondary memory, is the knowledge of a former state of mind after it has been dropped from consciousness. He continues to describe memory as being the knowledge of an event or fact that we have not been thinking about, but with the additional consciousness that we have thought or experienced it before. From his writings we can glean that he was very much aware of unconscious memory. His book, which took twelve years to write, was an immediate success and he became a leading psychologist of his day. It is still considered to be the most important text in the history of modern psychology and human thought. He then devoted his life to his other interests of philosophy and religion. It is to him that Pragmatism owes its fame as a movement in philosophy, having concern for the practical rather than for theories and ideals.

Sigmund Freud 1836-1939

Freud graduated from the University of Vienna Medical School in 1881. With his interest in nervous diseases and research into cerebral palsy with children, he became a lecturer in neuropathology at the university. In 1884 he had become interested in Breuer's treatment of hysteria by hypnosis, during which the patient was induced to remember their past.

Freud writes the word *primal* in a letter in 1897, but after his partnership with Breuer dissolved he took the decision to replace hypnotism by the method of *free association*. For more than ten years Freud stood completely isolated from the medical world with his theories either being completely ignored or ridiculed, as they were also controversial. As well as *free association*, his therapeutic techniques included the theory of *transference* in the therapeutic relationship and the interpretation of dreams. Eventually his work in psychoanalysis led to the establishing of the International Psycho-Analytic Association in 1910.

Freud believed many people repress painful memories into their unconscious mind. He attempted to find patterns of repression in patients to derive a general model of the mind. He believed people were unaware that they have buried memories or traumatic experiences and that repression did not take place within a person's consciousness.

Freud writes of *'primal repression'* as the *first phase of repression* in a paper entitled *Repression* in 1915. He advocates that repression is an element of avoiding pain—that a primal repression is the first phase of repression, which is a denial of entry into consciousness. He refers to *the second phase of repression* as *'repression proper'*, believing that the essence of repression lies simply in the function of rejecting and keeping something out of consciousness.

In his selected papers on Hysteria, Freud states his surprise when the individual hysterical symptoms immediately disappeared without returning:

"...if we succeeded in thoroughly awakening the memories of the causal process with its accompanying affect, and if the patient circumstantially discussed the process in the most detailed manner and gave verbal expression to the affect."

He also stated that recollections without affects are most utterly useless. The psychic process which originally elapsed must be reproduced as vividly as possible so as to bring it back into the *statum nascendi* (the condition of birth and then thoroughly *'talked out'*).

Early Freudian thought—that birth was the primal anxiety, and might be a traumatic birth—was a taster for the roots of birth psychology today. The dismissal of such notions and the almost total ignorance of life in the womb from Freud's contemporaries led to various persistent misunderstandings since then amongst psychoanalysts; the most profound of these being that memory cannot possibly go back as far as birth, let alone conception. Freud himself stopped short of believing there could be mental life active at birth, so when his patients had any type of birth memory he considered it to be a fantasy constructed by the mind at a later date, rather than actual memory.

Freud moved into his own self analysis by analyzing his own dreams. After publishing, *The Interpretation of Dreams* in 1900, he turned away from any contact with the primal process, away from the emotionally explosive abreactive cathartic method revealed in dreams, free association and transference. He saw these as secondary processes which could be subjected to rational analysis. He used the much more rational method of analysis which he named *Psychoanalysis*, rather than the other form of secondary process, repression of primal process. His new model was adopted by future psychoanalysts and this persists today, despite plenty of existing evidence to the contrary.

Joan Woodward, an English psychoanalyst and author of, *The Lone Twin*, writes about memory starting in the foetus around six months, which led her to believe that the loss of a twin during the third trimester could, for that reason, have significance for some lone twins.

Slow progress is being made by some psychoanalysts in acknowledging that memory may start earlier in the womb. Since the advent of three and four dimensional ultrasound imaging, the unborn baby can be seen to smile, frown, yawn, suck toes, feel fingers and interact with the womb environment much earlier than was ever thought possible.

Otto Rank 1884-1939

Otto Rank, in 1923, was one of the first people to seriously deal with the trauma of birth as being important for psychotherapy. Rank was a young friend and early associate of Freud, who encouraged his young protégé to pursue and develop his theory of birth trauma. When Rank first shared his manuscript, *Das Trauma der Geburt (The Trauma of Birth)* with Freud in 1923, Freud initially reacted to Rank's work as the most important progress since the discovery of psychoanalysis.

Rank stated that not only was birth the first experienced anxiety, but it was the prime source material for all the neuroses and character disorders speculating that the emotional shock was the underlying cause for all personality dysfunction. Rank wrote:

"We believe we have discovered in the trauma of birth the primal trauma."

He furthered this idea by continuing:

"We have recognized the neuroses in all their manifold forms as reproductions of, and reactions to, the birth trauma."

Rank went far beyond Freud in believing that virtually all psychological problems and human behaviour belonged to individual reactions to trauma at birth.

Freud later discarded the idea of birth trauma, also rejecting Rank himself, as Lake writes that Freud's contemporaries in-flamed his (Freud's) fear lest the whole of his life's work be dissolved by the importance attached to the trauma of birth. Freud feared that Rank's work would be a potential threat to his work on the Oedipus complex. Lake refers to Rank's belief that all symptoms ultimately relate to this primal fixation and that the place of fixation is in the maternal body and in perinatal experiences.

Freud's dismissal of Rank's work and his ideas on birth trauma seem to have adversely affected the course of psychoanalysis ever since. Rank's book is full of Freudian jargon and is not very easy to read, but it has some interesting material and is years ahead of its time.

After the publication of this book there was a period of misunderstanding of the nature of birth trauma. In 1928 Marion Kenworthy, a respected psychiatrist, tried to extend Rank's controversial theory in a paper entitled, *The Prenatal and Early Postnatal Phenomena of Consciousness*. She suggests that the emotional disorder known as *anxiety neurosis* is caused by psychological trauma which occurs at birth. Rank believed the womb to be a *'primal paradise'* which was lost by the separation at birth. Kenworthy said that the child born by Caesarian Section was prone to be less sensitized, cried less and was less irritated by contacts of handling than the baby delivered through the birth canal. She warned of profound nervous and emotional shock from every hard birth experience and encouraged obstetricians to keep pregnant women on diets to have smaller babies, who would then birth their babies through a birth canal without pain and trauma.

Rank himself took responsibility for some of this confusion, but his main work was psychological. He advocated that Caesarian birth had no way of preventing the separation from mother and trauma caused by this. Rank attempted to find ways to work directly with the primal process but was unable to develop a technique and finally moved away from primal process in his later career.

The development in obstetrics increased medicalisation of pregnancy. With more births taking place in hospitals at this time, this led to findings in the therapy room of psychological problems arising from medical and obstetrical intervention births. This trend is moving the other way now, thanks to the work of Michael Odent and Frederick Leboyer and many others, who are advocating birth without violence and more natural methods of delivery. The irony is that in some cases awareness of the trauma of birth has had the effect of making birth more traumatic for both mother and child.

Nandor Fodor 1895-1964

Nandor Fodor was a Hungarian journalist, attorney and psychologist who lived in England and America for most of his life. He was another contemporary with Freud who admired his work on spiritualism and psychic events, exploding the myth of the poltergeist.

Fodor was one of Rank's patients who became a psychiatrist, whose clinical work focused on the formative experiences of birth and the patient's emotional rebirth mainly through dream interpretation. Fodor's book, *The Search for the Beloved: A Clinical Investigation of The Trauma of Birth and Prenatal Conditioning*, was published in 1949. He really continues the search for prenatal wisdom and is another step towards the modern prenatal psychology movement. He wrote: *"God's laboratory on earth is the womb."*

Here are some other quotations from Fodor, which characterize the essence of Fodor's independent clinical claims. Some examples are:

"The greatest danger of injuries in early life is that they may mobilize and keep active the trauma of birth.

My finding is that every experience in suffocation tends to mobilize the buried memory of birth and that, ultimately, the fear of dying from loss of breath is a re-enactment of the panic which we drew our first lungful of air in this world. The unconscious mind tries to dispose of the trauma of birth by projecting it into the future in the form of death. Were we able to retrace our steps to the very source of life back to the mother's womb, we might find the answer to the mystery of our existence—at least we will not have this splendid illusion wrested from us. I believe that the degree of love which the new-born child needs is in direct proportion to the intensity of the trauma of its birth."

Lietaert Peerbolte in his book, *Prenatal Dynamics*, published in 1954, notes that Foder's investigations discovered two very important facts; firstly, that experiences at birth and in the prenatal state seems to be recorded and reproduced in dreams; and secondly, these experiences are apparently influencing postnatal psychical development. They form the base of several neurotic symptoms of the adult. Time and again people speak of dreams relating to contractions that feel like the swell and pull of waves on the seashore, and the swirl of the energy vortex and feeling of falling. It has been known that people end this dream by falling out of bed!

Francis J Mott

Mott was an English psychoanalyst who trained with Fodor. Again, it was through dreams that Mott developed a sense of the foetal life in the womb. He gave the world the idea of *Negative Umbilical Affect*. As we shall see, Frank Lake developed this idea, incorporating that of Mott on umbilical affect, positive and negative.

Lake's key to this research was the finding of, and confirmation by the work of F.J. Mott and according to Lake, other neglected psychoanalysts.

Mott also refers to changes in the method of oxygenation of the blood in the foetus. He describes that before birth the placenta oxygenates the blood, acting like a great gill, but at birth the lungs take over this function, so that oxygenation, which was formerly done outside the (foetal) body, is then done inside the (neonatal) body. Another example he gives of this reversal of function from outside to inside the body is that of the making of blood. At the beginning of embryonic life, when the circulation of the blood is initiated, the making of the blood is done in the placenta. After birth this is taken over by the bone marrow.

Mott was a Christian Scientist heavily into the total integration of creation. This resonates so well with the fractals idea that I incorporated it into the pre- and perinatal work in 1991, that Mott—as was Freud and Fodor—finding out that there were emerging patterns. For generations, the ideas of patterns and rhythms have been intuited and with the help of modern technology, foetal medicine and the studies of foetal development, they make total sense. These rhythms and patterns can be expressed using normal vocabulary with words like *'fractals'* becoming part of everyday language. What had been missing for generations was the word that described these rhythms and patterns.

Mott believed the laws governing the formation of the individual mind are identical with those which govern the development of that mind into its collective involvements. The principles governing the making of mind, both individual and collective, are identical with those which govern the formation of the atom, the solar system, the living cell and the metacellular organisms.

The patterns that Mott discovered through the Christian Scientists were identified as, *The Universal Design of Life*. When Frank Lake visited Francis Mott at his home he was distressed to be shown boxes of Mott's unsold books stored in the garage. Today, it is a rare phenomenon to find Mott's books. His findings are of such importance now that those unsold books could have been of great value to students of his work today.

Chapter 2

DR. FRANK LAKE

(1914–1982)

HIS LIFE AND WORK

Frank Lake - His Life, His Work

"The increasingly distressing, very real dangers, now being generated in present day wombs, and often forceps assisted or rapidly induced births we provide for babies, will ensure a steady supply of damaged adults, who will see it all just as we do and carry on the carnage." ~ Frank Lake

Frank Lake was an extraordinary man whose life was dedicated to understanding human suffering. I first met him in 1976 and feel privileged to have been associated with him and his work. It was only six years, but those six years filled me with the greatest hope anyone had ever given me for the future of the human race. Frank died in 1982 and, like many great pioneers and inventors, his work was not wholly recognised nor accepted during his lifetime. His enthusiasm and passion for the work rubbed off on me and midst other exciting experiences, I have continued to research, teach and develop his most stimulating and ground breaking work about life in the womb and its effect upon the adult personality.

I don't believe it would have been possible for Frank to see his projects and ideas come to fruition in his lifetime. They were immensely important for the future of the human race, to understand the early years of each individual life and the effect of conception, womb life and birth on child and adult behaviour. It was to take, and will take, many more years to be wholly accepted—but it is happening.

We now know, nearly forty years after his death, that not only those of us whom he mentored, but key figures in the work have come together worldwide and now totally agree that this part of our lives from conception to birth is the most influential in any person's life. Those who are sceptical may continue to be so, but Frank often threw the gauntlet down to his sceptics and challenged them to get down on the floor and experience what he was talking about. He also had the guts to experience for himself what he was talking about but in those days, he was the mentor and trusted few to work with him. He wrote extensively about the schizoid personality in his book, understanding it from experience, but having little success to heal his difficulties of staying close to people and being intimate with those who loved him.

This was the biggest criticism I ever heard about him, as he became close to clients and then vanished for weeks at a time on his travels.

The book written about him by John Peters, *Frank Lake: the Man and His Work* gives a one-sided account of his life. His family suffered greatly by this single-mindedness about his work. One particular loving paragraph by his daughter Monica stands out for me, as she cared for him in her Rushden home the weeks before he died:-

"The telephone seemed to ring constantly with relatives, friends and colleagues anxious to know how he was. I felt he was so greatly blessed to have the love and prayers of so many people. We received hundreds of letters and many beautiful flowers which filled his room with the fragrance of spring that he was missing outside. All this made me realise how much he must have meant to so many people and I felt privileged to be his daughter. I began to understand why, when sometimes in life a person has to give his 'all' to the world, he will have nothing left to give at home. There just isn't enough of him to go round. Sacrifices have to be made. At last I could learn to come to terms with and accept that my loss of a fatherly figure, presence and support meant a gain for hundreds of others."

Frank's search for answers to help others in their relationships did not benefit him in his lifetime but he laid the foundations for others to discover, and follow what he believed to be the roots of these debilitating characteristics of humanity. There are those who do not believe in self-sacrifice, seeing it as wasteful, perhaps self-indulgent, but whatever one's entelechy in life is, it asks us to give truly of our best with the gifts, talents and potential that we have. It is a choice, but for those with vision and genius that Frank had, the sacrifice does have to be made. It never goes without recognition in the long run, however many years it takes.

The Early Years

Frank was born in Aughton in Lancashire in the north west of England on June 6th, 1914, shortly before World War 1. Frank's brother Brian, born 1922, describes Frank's early childhood as being church-centred and how the three brothers, Frank, Brian and Ralph (born 1917), were expected to sing in the choir at Matins and Evensong, as their father was an organist and choir master. Frank attended the church school in the village and then went on to the High School in Liverpool that his father had attended. His mother Mary had been a teacher before her marriage and his father worked at the Liverpool Stock Exchange. They were simple Lancashire people and both were churchgoers from their early days.

A Medical Doctor And A Missionary

Frank went off to Edinburgh in 1932 and qualified as a medical doctor in 1937 at the age of 23. He also received some theological training there and at Selly Oak College, Birmingham. He rarely saw his family, but before he sailed for India, he met his future wife Sylvia at Swanwick Conference Centre in Derbyshire. They were engaged three weeks before, having qualified, he sailed to Bengal as a medical missionary in 1939. They were not to meet again for four and a half years.

It was his interest in theology and deep concern for human suffering that led him there. He stayed there throughout the Second World War, becoming an army commandant in Poona from 1941 to 1945, but Sylvia, experiencing her own adventures, landed in Bombay in 1944, met Frank again and married him three weeks later in Poona. Their son David was born in June 1945 in Poona. Sylvia experienced bouts of amoebic dysentery and when pregnant with their second child she returned home to Nottingham where Monica was born in 1946. Frank was not to see his wife and children for another fourteen months.

The long distances and time span in their relationship caused many difficulties and Frank's priority with his work and lecturing was always going to be reason for difficult family relationships. From 1946 to 1949 Frank was Superintendent of the Christian Medical College at Vellore, in South India and it was here that he ran the parasitology clinic from 1946 and became interested in psychiatry. In 1948 he returned to England for a long visit but in 1949 returned to India alone. Sylvia, pregnant with their third child Marguerite, stayed in England. On reading the sketch of Frank Lake's life in Peter's book the reader cannot fail to be moved by the almost impossible situation. Knowing his desire to remove suffering from humanity, which was Frank's life work, escalated his own family's pain and suffering.

At the same time he was one of the five founder members of the internationally acclaimed, Church of South India. Even in these early days of his career his interests and talents were wide and varied. He never lost his enthusiasm for India and often whilst having supper with him and Alison Hunter, who worked as a Pastoral Consultant with him, he spoke of the days in India and his early work there.

I was fascinated to listen to him, as at the time I was teaching the Church in the Modern World, for CSE students at Thomas Becket Upper School in Northampton and the Church of South India was part of the syllabus!

Into Psychiatry

Frank's meeting with Dr. Florence Nicholls who was Head of Psychiatry at the Christian Medical School in Madras must be mentioned here. He wrote:

"My first contact with dynamic psychiatry and with a psychoanalyst enlarged for me the dimensions of medicine. It now had to include a variety of imponderable emotional factors which I had never been taught to think about seriously before."

This meeting with her and her work transformed his life. His Christian background was fundamental to his distinctive theological, medical and psychiatric explorations and research throughout his life.

Lake returned to England to study psychiatry and for the rest of his life it became his dominant interest. He spent a year at the Lawn Hospital in Lincoln (1951-52) and a further six years at Scalebor Park Hospital in Burley, Yorkshire (1952-58), where he studied for the Diploma in Psychological Medicine awarded by Leeds University. The family stayed put in Lincolnshire and moved to Ilkley in 1954. During this training, a psychotherapeutic approach was expected and time given for experiential investigations. He believed his real education in psychodynamics began in 1954 with the introduction of the abreactive agent LSD 25 into the therapy of neuroses and personality disorders and this will be discussed later.

His training was influenced by psychoanalytic ideas, and in particular, *the object-relations theory*, which he constantly sought to integrate into his work as his ideas developed. He was very concerned about the distress of clergy who were not trained to cope with emotional distress among their parishioners and they were often desperate with little or no support.

The Clinical Theology Association

In 1962 Frank Lake established the Clinical Theology Association, which embarked on post-ordination training of clergy in pastoral care and counselling in a way that created wider frontiers for the church. This was at a time when counselling was in its infancy as a profession and mostly took place as an informal adjunct to the work of the clergy. He initiated training nationally, which soon extended across the professions and denominations, with international connections.

Frank himself wanted to serve the home mission and help the clergy not only in their personal lives but also with the pastoral lives of their parishioners. He found over the length and time of his own training that many clergy had their own problems with no-one to turn for help. Their limitations from their own seminary trainings meant they were not equipped to listen or guide their own parishioners with their deepest concerns and problems. His book published in 1966 became the foundation for seminars offered in eleven diocesan centres and many clergy attending found them life changing.

The late Reverend Doctor Tony Gough from Leicester was part of a peer group that Alison Hunter founded in the late 1970's. He wrote to me and had this to say about these early days:-

"I first met Frank Lake in 1961 as part of my Post Ordination Training in the Diocese of Portsmouth. All the sprog curates gathered thinking this was just another lecture on pastoral approaches and how to get people into their churches. How wrong we were! Frank appeared as a diminutive pixie figure, totally unselfconscious, and proceeded to fire us with his own enthusiasm about what we came to know as the Dynamic Cycle of Life. I was immediately 'hooked' and could see how his analysis applied to my own life. I was certainly going round the Cycle the wrong way, attempting to obtain acceptance through achievement.

The Bishop of Chelmsford, some years later invited me to enroll for Frank's Seminars on Clinical Theology. During this time, I got to know Frank well, and was impressed with his openness to new ideas, especially those arriving from America-Gestalt Psychology, Transactional Analysis and (his own obsession) Primal Integration. There was no doubting his genius, but I believe this came at a price—he could be incredibly empathic when working with clients, while at the same time insensitive to the needs of others outside a clinical setting.

For example, I talked with Frank when my first marriage was falling apart, and his response was to ask me to let my wife know that she could approach him at any time! I felt he had passed by on the other side."

The two areas of Frank's work were developing from his interest in psychiatry—firstly, the seminar work with clergy and his passion for primal integration and secondly, his continuing research in the area of the development of the psyche from the experience of birth and later pre-birth memories.

Beginnings Of Prenatal Psychological Research

During the 1950's, some psychoanalysts were suggesting that the prenatal state may not have always been uniformly calm and relatively undisturbed, as generally believed. The idea was also emerging that unpleasant experiences during the prenatal stage might foreshadow later bad experiences during or after birth. In other words, it was being posited that some kind of prenatal, mental life might actually exist but the proving of foetal consciousness was the actual block to this hypothesis.

Lake himself admits that his real education in psychodynamics began in 1954 when the abreactive agent LSD-25 was introduced into the therapy of the neuroses and personality disorders. As his patients came week after week, he began to write down whatever the patients said under the influence of the drug when the memories of the unconscious mind emerged into consciousness. He learned that they were remembering events from the very first year of life. It appeared to him that the infant responded to the appearance or *connection* with the mother and where this was missing, the painful absence of the mother's *love* caused great distress to the infant. At first, what appeared to him and to some of his clients to be birth memories, he started to interpret differently as an analyst from the object relations standpoint, and focused on the relationship between mother and child, but soon a new truth became apparent. His research showed that the roots of neurotic conflict and deprivation almost invariably occurred much earlier than birth.

"What I was not prepared for was the frequent abreaction of birth trauma. I was assured by neurologists that the nervous system of the baby was such that it was out of the question that any memory to do with birth could be reliably recorded as fact...

But then a number of cases emerged in which the reliving of specific birth injuries, of forceps delivery, of cord round the neck... and various other dramatic episodes were so vivid, so unmistakable in their origin, and afterwards confirmed by the mother or reliable informants that my scepticism was shaken.

Even if the patient had known this or that difficulty had attended his entry into the world, nothing would convince him or her that this was a fantasy, and not an actual reliving of a vividly remembered birth. It seemed that Otto Rank had been right all along. This left me free to allow my patients to continue my education."

Lake then attended a European Conference with other people, including Stan Grof, who were experimenting with LSD in psychiatry and they were also recognizing birth trauma in their clients. He was told that it was the job of the neurologists to explain how it happened —but people really were reliving their births. He returned home and began listening and recognizing the validity of birth trauma and birth memories arising in his clients.

Exploring Birth Trauma

During the earlier years he was working with clients on the time of their stressful pregnancies or traumatic births. Through his research with over 1200 professional and lay people, he believed that he had proved that prenatal catastrophes are of major significance in the origins of psychosomatic disorders, the whole range of personality disturbances, behaviour problems and emotional trauma. What seemed to be occurring just didn't make sense to him as a conventional analyst. His clients appeared to be reliving their birth trauma but he had been taught that memory before three years old was just not possible.

For a time in the 1950's Lake began to use LSD-25 for clients within the therapeutic setting. He noticed, as Grof and others have done, that well over half of his fifty-eight patients, whilst under LSD, described experiences as if they were reliving events in the womb, birth or the first year of life. He gave LSD to the patients whom he considered might benefit from it and then would sit down beside them for hours just to see what came up. He would write it all down by hand, because in those days he had no tape recorder.

LSD was banned in the United Kingdom at the end of the 1960's and Lake then realised the value of Wilhelm Reich's Bodywork and also Bioenergetics techniques. He discovered that deeper breathing alone was a sufficient catalyst for people to remember their births.

Lake considered the more natural method of deep breathing as being far superior to LSD, as LSD tended to bring into consciousness areas of pain, trauma and material that the client was not ready for. He wrote that the pattern of deep breathing used naturally actually produces the theta rhythm activity in the brain, like biofeedback, in order to retrieve repressed emotions and memories.

He then realised that the memory of the trauma of birth and events surrounding it had affected the personality development of that person. Lake was one of the first psychiatrists in England to recognise the relevance of birth trauma in the development of personality and other personality difficulties. Lake knew that he was going against the norms of his training as a psychoanalyst but followed his own intuition. He wrote:-

"Now when some Freudians are implicitly critical of the master, by taking birth and maternal bonding seriously, we have had to push further back still and follow the intuition opened up to us by 'deep sea' fantasy journeys and recognise that life in the womb is a potent source of psychopathology."

When I met Frank in 1976, he was producing his best work. My greatest joy was his enthusiasm and his ever-generous sharing of his ideas whenever we met, which was usually every week. He often opened the door at Lingdale, if he were not working, as he had no receptionist, only a very patient secretary, Hope Le Sueur.

Usually he was clasping a clip board with the latest chart he had devised. His ideas flowed thick and fast and he always wanted to share what his latest ideas and hypotheses were, while asking questions and wondering what opinions and experiences I may have on the topic in hand. Sometimes he didn't open the door, but someone else usually did, but Frank was in the kitchen with a body being rebirthed through the legs of the kitchen table!

One day a workman passed by the door of the big room when it suddenly burst open and a head first birthing took place through the door with Frank not far behind as the midwife! Those were the days! When he found himself up against a boundary fence, he always went beyond it. He was always expanding onto the next area of knowledge, coming to the edge and pushing himself that next step further.

Exploring Birth Memories And Earlier

In our conversations, Lake often emphasised that although there was ample earlier evidence in the work of Nandor Fodor and J.F. Mott, he had not realised until 1970 how severely painful and well-remembered is the much earlier invasion of the foetus by maternal distress. Step-by-step and patiently with his clients, he tested his intuition and hypothesis to assist them in making their retrospective journey, and to develop techniques of contextualizing these primal experiences in the successive months of pregnancy. He states:

"We find we must begin at conception, through the blastocystic stage, to implantation and the events of the first trimester. It is here, in the first three months of life in the womb that we have encountered the origins of the main personality disorders and the psychosomatic stress conditions. Summarising findings in over one thousand two hundred subjects who have relived the intra-uterine journey, we have concluded that there exists what we have called the Maternal Foetal Distress Syndrome."

He hypothesised that when the mother-to-be was distressed in any way, the distress went straight through the umbilical cord to the developing foetus. The response to the foetus was two-fold: one was to experience distress because of the mother's distress, the other was its own distress in having to survive the mother's distress. He always highlighted two elements—one being the invasion of the foetus by the mother's often complex emotions and the second, the foetal response.

Lake developed this hypothesis firstly by working with adult clients whose mothers had experienced a difficult and distressing pregnancy. He believed that all the mother's feelings towards the baby came through the cord. These feelings might include love and acceptance, but may also include total disinterest and rejection. As by the 1970s there was a general understanding of the effect of stress hormones on individual emotional response, he was already aware that under stress catecholamines actually come through the cord to the foetus. He believed they also transmitted the mother's emotions about the pregnancy from within her own system, to her child.

He came to believe that the behavioural reactions of a pregnant mother affect her foetus in ways that contribute to its perceptions of itself and its womb environment and these perceptions persist into adult life.

As each pre-born baby is unique, he believed the negative stuff was pushed to different parts of the body depending, as we now think, on the part of the body being developed at the time the trauma came in, as well as the individual's own reaction.

In his intra-uterine research work the two major components were: The Maternal Foetal Distress Syndrome, or Negative Umbilical Affect and secondly the Dynamic Life Cycle.

The Maternal Foetal Distress Syndrome

I believe, amongst all his intra-uterine research work, that the major component was the Maternal Foetal Distress Syndrome, or Negative Umbilical Affect. Lake produced privately circulated research papers which included his important work on The Maternal-Foetal Distress Syndrome and The Existence and Manifestations of Umbilical Affect, Positive and Negative, Direct and Indirect.

To the uninitiated, this simply means that the foetus in the womb is invaded by the emotional states of the pregnant mother. Lake states that the emotional chemistry circulating in the mother's blood stream, which conveys her response to her own life situation as she perceives it to her own body, is transferred at the placenta into the umbilical and foetal circulation. If for example, she is fulfilled and joyful in response to friends, or full of hatred and bitterness at the horror and evil in the world, the baby is also transfused by these feelings. Lake's key to these research studies was the finding of, and confirmation by the work of F. J. Mott and others. Lake continued with his work, incorporating that of Mott on umbilical affect, positive and negative. His very simple model showing positive and negative reactions of umbilical affect are:-

A positive affect:—*the Foetus responds to the flow of the feelings of mother's positive aware attention, giving emotional regard, a sense of continuity and union and good feelings.*

A negative affect:—*The foetus has no feelings of recognition of its existence. No attention is given, no contact made and the foetus may respond to the mother's call for help.*

Strongly negative affect:—*Mother's reactions of hostility, fear, anxiety, disgust, aversion or bitterness; mother's hostility for being pregnant and longing for a miscarriage, planning and attempting abortion.*

This highly simplified scheme shows the underlying pre-birth affect that lies behind childhood behaviour disturbances, adult emotional difficulties and relationship disharmonies.

The Dynamic Life Cycle

This was a major component of his work. Lake was referring to the dynamics of the early mother-child relationship. He dared to put this mother-child bonding further back—to the feelings of mother at the actual birth of her baby and to the nine months in the womb. Lake explained the basic model as funded on Acceptance, Sustenance, Status and Achievement.

However, it is important to add that these four components are the healthy, normal dynamics of human behaviour. If we are accepted in the early stages of conception, pregnancy and birth we live this life cycle the correct way round, leading to a strong sense of status and identification. If not most of us reverse this and spend our lives achieving to be accepted, causing rejection, depression and sadness in our relationships. It may be the foundation for so much depression based on the original lack of acceptance by mother.

During pregnancy a loving, bonding relationship between mother and child arises if the mother accepts her unborn baby and the baby responds. From this an early bonding is formed. If the communication of supplies, sustenance and care is positive on all levels of being, the bond is strengthened further. Lake believed that the status of the individual is already forming here; that the foetus knows what it is to-be-as-part-of-others and also to-be-as-oneself-alone. This strong sense of status and identification motivates a movement to give out to others. Lake stresses that the achievement is the actual output of what has been learned. This leads to personal being and a sense of well-being in the world of other people and things, leading to constructive activity in play, in gaining skills, in work and in human relationships.

Trauma In The First Trimester And Before

Lake's work became a cause of controversy among other analysts in the late 1970s. He proposed that the focus for psychopathology lay not in the field of Object Relations, where the emphasis on childhood development was focused on the quality of the first two years of the maternal-infant relationship life, but even earlier, in pre-birth life, particularly in the First Trimester, or the first thirteen weeks after conception. It was here that he also dared to take the baby/mother bonding back to the earliest possible time.

It was clear to him that the origin of every trauma does not lie in birth, but rather in the experiences of a foetus during its first three months, beginning with conception. Even the way the parents react when they find out they are expecting a child creates the environment in which an ovum is fertilized and will develop. In this way, the earliest experiences form a fundamental imprint of trauma, which persists throughout life.

In the later years of his life, Lake was working in a very new field of work. He was pioneering in England, and other countries, research studies, on traumas in the womb, especially in the first three months from conception, and their profound effect upon later patterns of life. He believed that these traumas caused negativity and disharmony in an individual, causing behaviour problems, and emotional disturbances, which possibly then caused learning difficulties. The crux of this research highlights the significance of the mother's emotional experiences early in pregnancy; that the foetus shares fully in the experience of the mother and her physical and mental and spiritual response to them. The unavoidable conclusion to this research was that :

These primal traumata, and so the origins of psychosomatic and personality disorders, were reliably attributable to displacement and containment of foetal distress during the first three months of life in the womb.

He spoke about these theories in lectures and conducted special workshops, which could bring about the recollection of buried memories as far back as the eight-day, blastocystic phase after conception.

He was convinced that the following were found by adults reliving those experiences: distress in the womb; the Maternal Foetal Distress Syndrome; bearing another's grief; mental pain and physical anguish. He was sure he was finding the roots of major personality disorders.

Knowing where the present day adult trauma came from, he helped the adult to integrate and change behaviour patterns, heal emotional disturbances, and use more creative activity. It remained to be seen if this was accessible to therapeutic intervention by the process of primal integration. It was within this framework that Lake developed his ideas and skills. Primal integration was criticised because it is difficult to assess by scientific methods and was at risk of refutation if evidence did not support it.

Grof's Four Basic Perinatal Matrices

Part of primal integration is *Rebirthing*—where clients are taken through their own birth. People re-experience intra-uterine and peri-natal experiences in the course of re-birthing. Grof used LSD, to loosen the repressive *gating*, covering the pain of birth. In his classic study of 1975, Grof drew attention to four Basic Perinatal Matrices:-

Before birth
The beginning of labour, before the cervix opens
The struggle to get out
Having emerged, the baby starts to breathe and establishes a new existence

Lake extended this idea to include the whole time in the womb. This research was done experientially by re-birthing adults in a therapeutic situation, with people whose present life was blocked emotionally, which was causing behaviour disturbances and relationship difficulties.

He points out that if each positive stage of growth is not properly facilitated, an incomplete phase contaminates the next phase and therefore past-contaminated transitions contaminate present ones.

In other words, the character, behaviour and emotional disturbances worsen and the individual may become labelled as maladjusted, unteachable, delinquent or un-manageable.

Frank Lake developed his theory, that if one phase is botched up the problem is carried onto the next phase, from Erik Erikson's work, which divided human life into eight stages. Lake simply added a ninth stage—from conception to birth. Being the synthesizer he was, he took Erikson, Piaget and Grof and put them altogether with his own theories and hypotheses.

Lake's Method Of Working

Lake used large cushions and blankets to enhance the awareness of the womb and then developed a guided fantasy, which reflected as accurately as possible the stages of development of the embryo from ovulation on, to about the stage of the third month of pregnancy. A surprisingly high proportion of people appeared to get in touch with personal experiences in the first trimester, which seemed to have some meaning and value for them.

Today, primal integration therapy is wide-ranging and eclectic but basically it involves a process of recapitulation and assimilation. That is, the client re-experiences the original trauma and then is able to assimilate this into consciousness, after which there is no need to act out the trauma in present day life.

Having experienced primal integration therapy myself, I have relived my own traumas in my mother's womb and the horrific birth that followed. As a result I have been able to recognise and try to change my behaviour patterns. Although superficially it appeared that I was OK, deep down, I experienced an inner life of misunderstanding and conflict, which my developed behaviour patterns were able to mask and block from awareness. However, it was much later in life, that by achieving more knowledge, and a situation concerning my mother's impending death, that I have been able to experience the deeper, more damaging events that scarred my personality. I know that I am still learning to communicate far more positively in deeper relationships and trying to achieve greater self-confidence rather than deep seated insecurities. I am acquiring a better self-concept and no longer need to project negative transference onto life, although this is something so many of us find difficult.

One of the greatest things to realize with this work is that where there has been extensive trauma in the prenatal period instant healing is not possible. At various times in life when traumatic situations arise they may take us into the early traumas that still need healing. I don't believe there are many of us, if any, who escape some type of birth associated trauma. But we can still work on achieving the best possible birth situations for our children's children.

Meeting Frank Lake

There were many people who met Frank during his life time, who benefited greatly from sharing a few hours with him. One of these people was Father Derek Lance, a Catholic priest from the Northampton Diocese who writes of his personal experience with such a meeting in the mid 1970's:-

Smell The Roses

The first sight I had of Frank Lake was of him smelling the roses in the garden of Mount Saint Bernard Cistercian Abbey, Coalville, Leicestershire. I didn't know him then. I thought this very ordinary figure, peering over his half—moon spectacles, totally absorbed in appreciating the rose, was just a fellow guest at the monastery. I don't think I had even heard his name before Fr Bernard pointed him out to me and I certainly knew nothing of his reputation, qualifications or writings.

When Fr Bernard explained that Frank had written that big book, 'Clinical Theology' it didn't interest me. I felt that the last thing I needed was a book on Theology, even Clinical Theology, whatever that could mean. Later I came to realise that what I desperately did need was to meet Frank Lake and to experience his healing therapy.

I had come to Mount Saint Bernard's for a rest and to get away from the unbearable situation in the parish where I was a priest. After a very successful career in teaching and with an international reputation as a lecturer and writer on Religious Education, at the age of forty-three I had been ordained a Catholic priest. I thought that now, with ordination all would unfold. But in my first two years as a priest it was as if it all folded up! There were moments of joy in my new ministry, but only moments. The predominant sense was of misunderstanding, rejection, isolation and depression. I had been sent to a parish where I had lived my childhood. The presbytery, Victorian Neo-Gothic, had a heritage plaque reading, 'Site of Norwich Prison'. That's what it felt like.

I was often depressed and at one time oppressed by crazy suicidal thoughts. I lost confidence in my priesthood and in myself. I even enquired about the procedure for leaving the priesthood. There seemed to be no help from advice and Confession failed to root out the resentment and anger in my heart. There seemed no way out.

Thus I came to Mount Saint Bernard and saw Frank smelling the roses. The next day I happened to be next to him at breakfast and, in answer to persistent questions of another guest, Frank explained his therapy of rebirthing and helping people to recover the memories of prenatal experiences and thus to find understanding and healing. This interested me as I had come across prayer for healing of memories.

So later, I talked with Frank about his theories and therapy and mentioned very briefly something of my painful parish experience. Frank seemed immediately to tune in intuitively. He was more interested in me than theories. With a few perceptive questions he learnt from me that I had suffered from atopic eczema as I said, 'All my life since birth'. 'Not just since the time of your birth but because of your birth' he replied. Then I told him that the only two things I had been told by my family about my birth were that when I was born I didn't breathe and the doctor had given me up for dead and I survived only because of the persistence of a woman helper. 'It is not just that you didn't breathe; it's because you wouldn't breathe', Frank commented. The other thing was that my mother had been extremely ill at my birth and for a considerable time afterwards. So I must have been separated from her when I most needed her. It is interesting to recall now how quite often when people have offered me help, sympathy, or even love, I have responded, 'It's all come too late now.'

So Frank tentatively offered to help me experience this therapy of rebirth and recovering and reliving the intra—uterine memories and I accepted at once. Later that afternoon the session, if that's the right word, took place in a spare room in the monastery and Frank said all we needed was floor space, lots of pillows and lots of tissues. Fr Bernard and Fr Luke asked to be present and said they would be just there and pray silently. The session took about two hours and there isn't space here to describe it in detail. At one point, grinding my teeth, clenching my fists and feeling the most intense anger, I growled, 'I want to come out!'. Then I wanted to be touched and then couldn't bear to be touched. At another time I said, 'I'm my own space' and then, 'I'm dead. No, I am more than dead. I'm like water poured out on the ground.' I didn't realise at the time that this is a quotation from psalm 22, a psalm of dereliction that begins, 'My God, my God, why have you forsaken me... I call all day, my God, but you never answer.'

Then, involuntarily, I lay on my back, arms outstretched, ankles crossed and my mouth wide open and dry while tears poured down my cheeks. A perfect image of the crucifixion. Those familiar with Frank's work will recognise here maternal-foetal distress syndrome and schizoid position and personality.

I knew nothing of these terms then, but the experience I had of them was most real. My meeting with Frank Lake had been pure chance and coincidence. I believe it was providential. There was another coincidence. When immediately after, I joined the monks for Vespers, the first psalm just happened to be that same Psalm 22.

All I can say is that this therapy and prayer be Frank and the two monks really effected a radical healing. I felt the resentment lift from me and I was able to pray with tears, prayers of deep forgiveness.

People ask, 'What do you think of Frank Lake and his theories and therapy?' All I know is that my meeting with Frank and experiencing his therapy is undoubtedly the most important meeting in my entire life. It, he, saved my vocation, my sanity and my life.

Derek also spoke to me of his meeting with Frank's wife, Sylvia, who came to pick Frank up from the monastery. They met in the car park and Sylvia was most displeased to hear that Frank had worked with Derek. How did you stop a man from doing the work that he lived for?

The Three L's

The late Dr. John Rowan has been at the forefront of the Human Potential Movement since 1969 and was a founder member of the Association of Humanistic Psychology Practitioners. In 1972 he was Chairperson of the Association of Humanistic Psychology in Great Britain and in 1978 became Vice President of the European Association of Humanistic Psychology. John has been a good friend and Patron of Amethyst since its inception in 1982. He is a prolific writer, practices primal integration and was trained by the late Dr. William Swartley.

I asked John if he had any memories of Frank. He responded that he had not met Frank on a personal level but he had an interesting memory of him. In the late 1970's some time, there was a session in a hall in London where there were three L's on the stage together— Ronnie Laing, Frederic Leboyer and Frank Lake. Leboyer had just been attending one of Frank's 5-day workshops, where several people had re-experienced their birth. Someone asked Leboyer, who had apparently attended some 10,000 births, whether the re-experienced births were genuine or just imaginary reconstructions. He said that he had been very interested and had conducted several tests on the participants to find out the answer. One was the Babinski reflex, where newborn babies have a quite different response to that of an adult— these participants gave the neonate version and not the adult version.

Another was the Moro reflex, which again can distinguish between one and the other, and again the response was that of the newborn, not of an adult. This made a big impression on me (and, I think, others in the audience) and rather confirmed my belief that re-experiencing can be genuine and believable.

Hidden Springs

In the summer of 1978 there appeared on the scene, from Canada, Barney Pritchard, a therapist. Barney's story with Frank is as follows;

Between the years 1956 and 1968, we at Hidden Springs, a Christian rehabilitation centre, located in Paris, Ontario, Canada, received regular journals from Dr. Frank Lake at Lingdale, Nottinghamshire, England. I had helped to establish this centre as an assistant to the Rev Ralph Gordon Howlett, the Director, and was an active member of the staff of Hidden Springs for ten years.

I distinctly recall, in fact, possess a copy of one of these journals, entitled "The In Group and the Out Group in a Hospital Setting." It was a thorough study of the conflicts commonly experienced working in a hospital. These journals were valuable to us as we were pioneers in setting up this Residential Therapeutic Community. Ralph Howlett went to England on one occasion to meet Frank Lake.

In 1977 I had just returned from Campbell Hot Springs where Leonard Orr had set up a "rebirthing centre." I was keen to know more of this intriguing phenomena and I knew that Frank Lake was the world's authority on this subject. In February 1978 I found Frank's address and phone number and immediately phoned Lingdale. They told me that Frank Lake and William Emerson were holding a week long seminar in England in May 1978. I said, "I will be there!" This seminar was to examine first hand "The Perinatal Stage of Development of the Human Foetus", meaning before, during and after birth, and how that period of time affects us as adults.

This seminar was well led by William Emerson but Frank Lake was unable to attend as he had recently suffered a slight stroke. Upon completion of the seminar I proceeded to Lingdale and was given a room in the annexe. The garden at Lingdale badly needed help so I pitched in and did the obvious. Soon after that I met Frank and was able to book some private sessions. Frank was the expert and was very authoritative and professional and he also showed great care and compassion.

During one session I relived the moment when my mother realised she was pregnant. The shock was so great that I said, "I disappeared." These sessions were very useful to me and helped fill in a lot of "holes." During a further session I ended up reliving my own conception, with a very clear knowledge that this was a traumatic time for my mother especially. I remember debating whether to be created and born and finally deciding,

"Yes, I want to be created." Then following a lull and a voice above said quite clearly, "Oh, by the way, one more thing, just don't expect an easy life." As Frank recovered he was leading a birthing seminar and invited me to assist him. This was quite an honour and it all went well. During Frank's convalescence from his slight stroke his staff encouraged him to take a holiday. I said to him, 'Frank why don't you and I take a trip up to Scotland?' As usual Frank was in a hurry and drove like a rally driver. In fact, I have a picture in my mind's eye of a fairly slight man, armed with a clip board and his half glasses, moving around Lingdale with a twenty degree bend from his waist down and always in a hurry.

After a few days we arrived at Findhorn in Scotland—a spiritual community. Frank was well-known and respected. From there we proceeded to Iona and we stayed in the Founder's Quarters on Iona—very posh too! We attended a Scottish ceilidh which I thoroughly enjoyed. I suspect Frank would judge this to be somewhat of an indulgence! One evening I arrived in our quarter to find Frank conducting a full-blown rebirthing session. Perhaps this was indicative of the perpetuation of the "protestant ethic" which implies "work = salvation." He just could not get free from his work. We also visited the Isle of Skye and many favourite and wonderful places, where Frank had spent many holidays with Sylvia and their children.

In due course we arrived back at Lingdale in time for Frank's birthday. All in all it was an excellent trip and I shall continue to cherish the memories.

Barney saw Frank as being extremely committed to his purpose in life, the intra-uterine research and also being a very committed Christian fundamentalist. He believed Frank was trying to bring about a marriage between science and religion, and maybe he was one of the early pioneers of the 20th century trying to do this. Although his last years were spent helping people regress to their primal time in the womb Barney believed he drew a line there and to his knowledge never supported reincarnation or other life times.

Frank Lake's Legacy

Lake's book *Tight Corners in Pastoral Counselling* had a very mixed reception, in the heat of which he was dying of cancer. Inevitably, this brought about both positive and negative reactions, in which Lake was fully engaged. He was also trying to complete a paper entitled *Mutual Caring*, which was edited and retitled *The First Trimester* by David Wasdell. Frank's death in 1982 brought the discussion to an end. The world was robbed of his genius in the work, but he left a great legacy for others to continue his work more unobtrusively; and this is what we have done in Amethyst for over twenty five years. In response to his critics, Lake himself is essentially reassuring when he writes:

In no sense do these discoveries of prenatal components in the health and sickness of the human person, invalidate existing knowledge about genetic, hereditary and constitutional factors, nor do they negate what is known about the effects of birth itself and post natal and childhood psychodynamic interactions. They do add a hitherto neglected dimension.

This, I believe, needed to be said, as when new concepts such as Lake's are brought forth, many professionals may become threatened that their own ideas are obsolete and incorrect. This is not so, and Lake himself is the first to give reassurance on this point. He wrote:

...the great danger is that, as many times before, we will interpret the fact of recession, on whatever scale or level it affects us personally, by evoking similar patterns of conflict and response from the past, that is, by regression. If this happens, it will be a regression, not to post-natal human levels of experience, but to pre-natal first and third trimester levels, of constrictions, threatening pressures, confused internal states and pollutions and to similar patterns derived from even more crushingly frightening births. All these regressions belong to pre-personal levels, indeed to impersonal conflicts and resolutions.

Lake was seeing the possibility of what is happening world-wide now. He impressed upon his readers that we would confront each other, locked in impersonal blocks of force and counter force, constricting and being constricted, polluting and being polluted, suffocating and being suffocated. Yet we would all feel quite justified in our fantasy-based cruelties, reacting to our fantasy dangers, because they would, upon regression, be derived from impressions stored in pre-natal memory.

Chapter 3

THE AMETHYST RESOURCE FOR HUMAN DEVELOPMENT

Worldwide Developments In Primal Therapy

Amethyst was founded by Alison Hunter in 1982. Alison discovered prenatal psychotherapy as a result of working as a pastoral consultant with Frank Lake at his Clinical Theology Centre from 1976-79 and became very interested in his work. We began running workshops there together in 1978, and in Northern Ireland as well as England.

In 1970 Arthur Janov, published his book *The Primal Scream: Primal Therapy-The Cure for Neurosis.* The International Primal Association (IPA) was founded in 1973 by a group of therapists working with *'primal'* material. In the teeth of regular scathing attacks by the scientific community, primal therapy and its accompanying ideas about the nature of early consciousness was developing rapidly in the 1980s, all over the world.

By this time, in Australia Dr. Graham Farrant (1933-1993), an eminent Australian child psychiatrist was also doing pioneering work on pre- and perinatal trauma. He had discovered primal therapy for himself in a session with Janov in 1973. At that time he was already sure that his patients were remembering their birth, which at the time Janov would not accept. He moved to the Denver Primal Centre until he returned to Melbourne and set up the first primal therapy centre in Australia at Erin Street in Richmond. During three-hour groups, clients would be taken through various levels of regression. In a further effort to reduce birth trauma, in 1976 at the Queen Victoria Hospital in Melbourne he instigated a gentler birthing process in order to reduce the traumatic effect on the new-born of noise, bright lights, rough handling and separation from mother.

Another pioneer was William Emerson, another member of the IPA who spent a good deal of time in Europe. He had been trained as a clinician, and worked for some time in hospitals, but got more and more involved with regression and integration therapy. He also started calling his work, *Primal Integration.*

In the early 1980's our work at Amethyst was influenced by William Emerson's research; and also the introduction into Ireland of Reichian and Bioenergetics techniques and holistic therapies.

Our work developed rapidly in helping clients relive their conception, womb and birth experiences.

Frank Lake's hypothesis was that any trauma happening to the pregnant mother was passed to the foetus through the umbilical cord. We found that clients were experiencing, as a foetus, being marinated in the negativity of a particular trauma. The personality and character developed similarly. So not only would the foetus experience trauma through the umbilical cord, but also by being wholly embraced within mother's auric field.

Working With Frank Lake's Ideas

In those days, we were working with Frank's early hypothesis that birth trauma set the pattern for personality development in life, and we still work with many people in this area. When Alison was working with Frank in the late '70s he was studying the maternal/foetal distress syndrome. This was because he was coming across so many people with distress that was obviously earlier than the birth trauma. He believed any trauma happening to the pregnant mother was passed on to the foetus through the umbilical cord. Out of that idea came another, more fundamental concept, which he wrote about in his final book. He felt there must be some kind of cellular memory spanning generations and coming into the sperm and the ovum at conception.

We decided to incorporate these new ideas of cellular memory into our work. As we continued our work it became clear that Frank Lake's untimely death was not going to put an end to the development of this extraordinary idea. Our way of working was to suggest that a client lay on a mattress on the floor with protective cushions around and if it felt right, to curl up in the foetal position. Concentrating on breathing more deeply, the client was able to contact feelings and go where body, mind and spirit needed to wander in order to explore where these early traumas lay. The healing seemed to happen when the client regressed to an early trauma and gained insight that the response of the foetus, the baby or the young child now need not be imitated in the adult's present day life. A change of behaviour could now occur, and the adult react in a rational way rather than that of the irrational child.

We understood there had to be three parts for a primal trauma to be healed: emotional feeling, physical sensation and historical memory. The whole process appeared unexplainable and for many clients, their negative approaches to life seemed irreparable and unhealable.

Wounded people suffered the degrading feelings of being unlovable, rejected, and often an insurmountable terror or dread of death. Their lives damaged, their feelings wounded, egos non-existent, these responses were transferred and projected onto people and situations. By reliving the birth process physiologically, psychologically and spiritually where negativity occurred, and by bringing this negative situation into consciousness, it seemed to facilitate the healing process and the negative reactions could be returned to the initial trauma.

Cellular Consciousness

Dr. Graham Farrant was himself the survivor of an attempted abortion, which he confirmed with his mother. He therefore emphasised the importance of parents being emotionally prepared for the act of conception. Later in his career as a child psychiatrist, he encouraged the exploration of the use of primal therapy in children and babies to heal birth and intra-uterine traumas.

His experience with regression led him to focus more on conception and implantation, he, like Lake, came to believe that memories were held at the cellular level—he called it *cellular consciousness*. He said:

Cellular memory refers to a kind of preverbal memory, contained within the physical body of experiences that occurred when we were gametes. That is to say, there is a body memory, a cellular memory, of our experience as a sperm, and also of our experience as an egg.

At Amethyst we were glad to see that Lake's ideas were gaining ground. From the start we have evidence that suggests that cellular consciousness, foetal consciousness and birth consciousness all exist, and have an effect upon the whole of life.

Past Life Therapy, Genetic Memory Or Ancestral Memory?

Our knowledge in this field of work is limited, curtailed by a negative and narrow Christian attitude towards reincarnation and the possibility of past lives. What we have experienced with clients and ourselves, on the therapy room floor, surely is the reliving of lives in the distant past.

For those who believe in reincarnation this is an everyday occurrence; for those who don't, many questions arise. There is the possibility of genetic memory, like something happening to an ancestor centuries ago becoming part of today's family and needing to be healed through a number of generations. This allows for the possibility of cellular and genetic memory.

The ovaries we come from were already in our grandmothers when our mothers were born. When our mothers were conceived by their mothers the ovaries were already there in grandmother. So, cellular consciousness carried by us, medically speaking, goes back three generations. This could be the cellular basis of ancestral memory. When one-to-one counselling does not achieve the required depth for change and transformation, then it is sometimes necessary to try and reach the root of the problem by counselling further back.

An Eclectic Approach To Therapy

Now we have entered into the twenty-first century, many people in varied professions are looking to synthesise a wide range of disciplines in order to find out the truth about our human condition. Whichever way the inner journey is facilitated for the client, to look at intra-uterine life, birth and neonatal and resolve any trauma that may lie there, is of absolute necessity if there is to be healing. Since the 1980s, pre and perinatal psychotherapy has become a recognised and widely practiced style of therapy. At Amethyst today, we use a wide range of therapies in individual and group therapy. We intend to continue to develop the work and ideas of Frank Lake. We also offer training to the pre- and perinatal psychotherapists of the future, so these ideas will remain current in years to come.

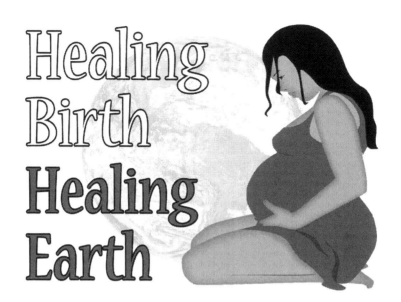

PART TWO

Chapter 4

BIRTH METAPHOR

Birth Metaphor

This chapter is my attempt to clarify some of those signs and symbols which may be overlooked, or even ignored, by people who do not have the vocabulary to describe them—most particularly the clients themselves.

Alongside our therapeutic work with individuals and groups, the proving of foetal consciousness and cellular memory is central to the authenticity of our work. We constantly seek to narrow the plausibility and credibility gap that exists, even among those working in the same field.

Meanwhile, therapists working experientially with the healing techniques of pre- and perinatal psychotherapy will continue to do so, knowing that deep inner changes occur after the causes for trauma in people's lives have been found and resolved. The first step is to identify the pre-birth story for each individual.

These particular reactions and metaphors have powerful and useful linking functions for the therapist, as he or she seeks to understand what may lie behind them, for they bring fragmented bits into a comprehensive single picture.

Metaphors are imagination in action, freeing or enslaving human beings. They may be hard to see at first; for many of our everyday actions and feelings usefully describe, with some of the most powerful metaphors in the human language, events at birth, extending back through uterine life, implantation, and conception itself.

If these metaphors arise in everyday language, we call them *scripts*. Our research data, gathered over many years, reveals how birth scripts become life scripts, and how problems can be identified as having roots in conception trauma, fallopian tube trauma, implantation trauma, threatened and spontaneous abortions, twin loss and maternal foetal distress.

Verbal Expression Of Pre-Birth Scripts

The commonest and easiest clue to prenatal influences is to be found in the way people verbally describe their life experiences. Prenatal experiences are not generally recalled by adults or children in ordinary day-to-day living, with specific pictures and auditory language memory. Those experiences occurred before the development of verbal language.

People express their birth feelings metaphorically. That is, they may hold specific irrational beliefs which they vigorously defend, or they may make repeated use of particular images when they speak. For example, birth language can be obvious as *birth scripts* in everyday conversation:

"I saw the light at the end of the tunnel."
"I just couldn't see a way out."
"It's just all too difficult—I can't find a way out."
"I'm in a dreadful place—I just can't stand it!"
"It drives me round the bend!"

Many of these scripts are an expression of negative life patterns or imprinting, which we discover in those people who were having life difficulties and have come into therapy for help. Some know and some do not know that their problems had originated at birth. The birth scripts evolving from traumatic experiences colour the human throughout life.

Over the years we have listened to the stories of hundreds of people, for whom the moment of birth formed an impression, which has controlled them subsequently from a subconscious level. Adults come to us at a time of personal crisis, for foetal distress and trauma at birth emerge at a time of illness, or great pressure. Stressful situations such as separation and loss can trigger memories of birth trauma, but too often the birth story is not recognised by those unfamiliar with *birth language*. We believe therefore that this is a language worth learning.

Inappropriately Strong Feelings

Many people come to us filled with extremely strong and difficult feelings that they know are inappropriate and which may at times be overwhelming. This is a common reason for people to seek therapy, but for some people these feelings cannot be fully explained or healed, despite many months or even years of therapy. It may be that a deeper explanation is required—perhaps these strong feelings are related to intra-uterine events and experiences. This would be worth tentatively exploring, to trace these feelings back to their origin in the womb.

Anger

It is a widely accepted psychological principle that pain produces anger. Since even the best births involve some pain, it is inevitable that all of us are left with a subconscious residue of primal anger. Numerous clinicians from various approaches have observed the imprints of birth trauma in the psychological dysfunction of their clients. We see anger is one of the many feelings left over from the turmoil of birth. It can disempower us from before birth—and we may respond in anger as children and adults.

Lake emphasises that, during delivery, the rage of the baby can increase to murderous heights as it struggles to survive. As it tries to get out, the baby must survive what feel like murderous pressures and totally unreasonable demands. It is infuriated at being pushed out, but at the same time as being held in tighter than ever, with no instructions as to which way to turn. Knowledge of this behavioural birth language is vital for counselling.

The *birth anger script* is lived out as a way to express the feelings that arose in delivery. In born life, birth anger may well lead to misperception and irrational, de-skilled responses. Anger is also acted out as highly emotional violence, controlled or expressed, which is another kind of language we must learn to interpret accurately. This is where the problems arise that may bring some people into therapy.

In the acting out of birth trauma, that same angry, aggressive, driving behaviour that gets some babies out of the birth canal can cause problems in adult life—too much aggressive anger may cause a person to die prematurely from overwork or make personal relationships difficult.

The violent behaviour of adolescent youths can be seen as expressing the prebirth feelings that once accompanied invasive birth trauma. The medical intervention of the forceps provokes a murderous rage within the baby, which may be concealed for many years into adulthood. An adult born in a severe forceps contraction delivery has been pushed too soon into something they are not ready for. This may cause severe depression with underlying murderous rage. Some experience being pushed *over the edge* accompanied by a feeling of helplessness.

It may also signal the invasive violence that penetrated the foe—tus in the womb, the violent penis which penetrated the womb in rape and invasion or the *violent* sperm invading the unreceptive ovum.

Anxiety And Fear

Unreasonable feelings of fear, anxiety and panic, when there has been no trauma in born life, can be understood as symptoms of post-traumatic stress disorder related to birth or life in the womb. For instance a child may be very nervous, impatient, very fearful of failure and become tense if he does not succeed immediately. An adult may feel paralysed by fear of movement. This level of fear can be totally disabling.

A Feeling Of Stuck-ness

Sometimes a client will come with a complaint that despite working on their birth and womb experience for some time, they still *'get stuck in life'*. This may mean we have to go back a little further in life to find the root cause.

"I get stuck. Even after all the birth and womb trauma work that I have done, I still get stuck in life. The feelings are right through me. I start things and then can't seem to finish them. I put a lot of energy into things. I have a lot of drive but I then stop and can't continue. It's completely irrational. It is certainly earlier than birth. It seems earlier than I have done before."

This feeling can be expressed in various verbal ways and it is worth taking these words seriously.

"I am unable to move on."
"I can't cope with change."
"I have been in shock for a long time."
"I feel frozen."
"I want to be free."

Erratic And Self-Defeating Behaviours

The other non-verbal language we have to learn to understand is expressed in specific behaviours. The story is told in action—or inaction. We see many clients who knowingly employ erratic or self-defeating behaviour. We have learned to understand this a bid to convey or make sense of a specific, difficult feeling. We know that our attitudes to ourselves in the world are reflections of the life we had before birth. Where there has been trauma, even very early in life, this can be the cause of behaviour problems.

Traumas experienced in clients do often come from childhood trauma. Many (more than we have ever realised) have their origins in the period around birth and intra-uterine experiences—and even further back, to conception and preconception. These can cause trans-marginal stress (that is, beyond the point of bearing) and dissociation, that may arise during the nine months of gestation in the womb. The bigger picture may include other personality disorders, relating to paranoia, hysteria, anxiety, narcissism, depression, phobias and addictions.

Suicide Attempts

A little-considered reason for suicidal feelings is some kind of birth or intra-uterine trauma. It is my belief that at any point during the conception, pregnancy or birth, where the pain of the single cell, the blastocyst, the foetus, the pre-born, is beyond the point of bearing, suicidal thoughts and tendencies take their roots.

I lived my life at a superficial level and the pain was well hidden. But at times when it surfaced and became intolerable I wanted to die. I first attempted suicide at the age of thirteen with an overdose of pills. At the time I had no idea why I had done this—but parental illness, my own physical pain and family financial pressures caused intolerable responsibilities that I was too young to deal with. I had thought about ending it all, many times. My own regression work as an adult took me to the earliest places in my life when I experienced the primal pain of rejection through attempted abortion, more than once, and the most horrific forceps delivery that felt like it was severing my head from my body. I had no idea that my therapy would take me into these places and I certainly had no knowledge that the human organism was capable of remembering so far back.

The chosen method of suicide can also be a signal. One client who overdosed on alcohol and aspirin at 16 as the first of many suicide attempts, eventually found an explanation:

My way of attempting suicide through overdosing on medication can be connected to my mother taking medication for her migraine and blood pressure whilst pregnant with me. I was recreating, time and time again through events in my life, my time in utero and birth trauma.

Relationship Difficulties

Many clients come to us with relationship difficulties, such as social isolation, the fear of intimacy or the inability to make a commitment to a long-term relationship. The loss of a twin as far back as the fallopian tube or in the first weeks can lead to the roots of commitment anxiety combined with the fear of separation and intimate relationships. Our task has been to facilitate ways to help clients become functioning human beings in intimate relationships and friendships.

I believe that integrating the work of childhood trauma, healing the inner child and the traumas that pre-date it, are vital when relationship dysfunction is still apparent. A deeper healing occurs when the roots of the trauma are brought into consciousness and the client has the insight (and facilitator) to find the event, sensations and emotions that caused the primal trauma.

A New Language

In twenty years working with pre- and perinatal material, we have learned to detect and diagnose the various signs of pre- and perinatal influences. This is like a new language we are learning to speak. One of the many reasons for writing this book is that any form of counselling would be enriched by recognising and understanding early and pre-natal experiences, both in everyday life and during therapeutic encounters.

Chapter 5

BIRTH TRAUMA IN THE ADULT

Birth Trauma Sets A Pattern

Frank Lake categorically believed that what happens to us as newborns and even as pre-borns has a profound effect on us for the rest of our lives. In our years at Amethyst we have found this to be true, and so have many other therapists throughout the world. This chapter will focus on the most widespread problem, and the one that was first noticed by Otto Rank in 1934 as a probable cause of neurosis and other psychological problems in the adult—birth trauma.

Birth trauma includes any physical injury sustained by a baby during birth and also the psychological shock of experiencing the delivery process. The amazing findings of those experiencing primal techniques to re-live early trauma, could have enormous implications for birthing and child-rearing practices. As Frederick Leboyer so earnestly taught some years ago, we need to move towards a gentler, less intrusive style of delivery. This idea has gained great respect and there has been obvious success for those who adopted his methods.

It appears that when the birth experience has been traumatic it sets a life pattern. In other words, at the moment of birth, people form impressions which control them subsequently from a subconscious level. A distinction does have to be made between the projection of mature experience onto the foetal infantile world, and the triggering into adult behaviour of negative anger, anxiety, and terror patterns from the associated infantile experience.

Our research with the different types of birth over the years has shown specific scripts with similar types of birth. We find that in many people the foetal distress and the trauma of birth are repressed and do not emerge into consciousness again until late adolescence, early adult life or even middle life.

They may emerge at a time of illness, or at a time of great pressure or stressful situations. The discovery that our basic, original injuries take place during embryonic and foetal life requires that healing needs to take place at this same deep level if it is to be radical and complete.

Different Types Of Birth Trauma

Birth is essentially traumatic. The obvious medical classified birth types includes: breech; caesarean; forceps; induction; premature; transverse lie; late; long labours; fast births; cord round neck, amongst others. Many of these births may be classified as *difficult* or *traumatic*. The birth scripts evolving from traumatic experiences colour the person's personality throughout life.

Listed below are various scripts that we have noted from clients who experienced birth trauma. It does not necessarily follow that every person experiencing a particular type of birth will have the same scripts. For each birth there are between twenty and thirty birth scripts —only a few are mentioned here.

Breech Birth

A breech birth is violence in the womb and the breech-born becomes the victim:

It's difficult to do things the right way round.
I look for solutions but I feel so insecure.
I'm different from everyone, so I just stop thinking.
I want to back out when under pressure.
I'm afraid of being wrong so I have difficulty speaking up.

Premature Birth

In his book *The Mind of Your Newborn Baby*, David Chamberlain states that babies are telling us that Special Care Baby units are theatres of violence. Babies arriving early find themselves in a surreal environment of needles, lights, incubators and monitors designed for physical life support, but not for emotional life support. The designers of these nurseries were not expecting newborn babies to have thoughts, feelings, or the perception of pain. In adult regression work, we find that most of our clients who were born prematurely were put into an incubator—this means that they also need to be re-born out of the incubator to dissipate the anger.

Angrily—I am here.
I need you.
I need to be touched.
Pick me up and hold me.
I feel Mother is angry with me.
When she is angry with me I always end up feeling I can't move.
I want to get out of here.
Out! Out! Please open the door.
I want my own space.

Forceps

The medical intervention of the forceps provokes a murderous rage within the baby, concealed often for many years into adulthood. An adult born in a severe forceps contraction delivery is pushed too soon into something they are not ready for and it may cause severe depression, with underlying murderous rage. Some have periods of being pushed *over the edge* and others may become hospitalised.

Let me out.
There's no way out.
Get out of my way.
Don't tell me how to do it. I'll do it my way.
Why can't people do things properly—they are all so incompetent.
I'll do it myself, it's safer.
Life is such a struggle.
I can't make it on my own.

Induction

Either because of foetal distress, for medical reasons, or staff shortages, a birth is artificially started.

I am not ready!
Don't push me, I feel helpless.
I don't know what to do.
I am missing out on something.
Why can't someone else do something?
I just can't get started.
Wait! I am not doing that until I am ready.

Near Caesarian Birth

After a long labour there is the decision to operate. An imprinting is anger—the nearly-born saying angrily:

Cut her! If they cut her open I could get out.
Nothing will ever match that fight. Cut her! Cut her!

Caesarian Birth

It is ironical that disciples of Otto Rank proposed that all children should be born by caesarian section to eliminate birth trauma. Jane English describes the effect of caesarian births

as not being limited in time to the removal of the baby from the mother. It continues for years—caesarians appear *unborn*, as if their births are still in process.

I was ripped out.
I felt cheated, angry and not really here.
I really was raging—I could have done it myself.

Twin Births

The first twin may be the expected one. Terror at being the second, unexpected twin causes lack of self-confidence, rejection, and second-class-citizen syndrome. The second twin in the womb may push and become the first born, while the twin who was meant to be first was forced to be second. This causes great confusion in relationships. The more dominant twin may be born second, having pushed out the quieter of the two in order to have space to *get out*. This may result in someone willing to be kicked around in life until they decide to change it. It can lead to victim syndrome, bullying and commitment fear.

There is a classic *Second Twin Syndrome* script. A twin born second often thinks of the older twin as better, brighter and the leader. The second twin will put up with things; feels they cannot do anything about their own position. The second twin will often have to wait for something to happen, as there is *something* in the way.

Often this script appears as the second twin usually knows ways out of difficult situations but feels unable to do anything about it. Other second-twin scripts are:

I'm not recognised.
I don't know where I come in.
They are not expecting me.
They have forgotten me.
I am insignificant.
I shouldn't be here.

This stimulates a life script of not being able to trust, and some anger about being left out. The second twin follows the older twin:

I took the easy option and let him do it!

The first twin may have some guilt about the second twin but is also the leader. He or she often acts as the older brother or sister. Twins often want their own space. They have a fear of closeness, but also want it, and feel they cannot survive without the other.

Twin Loss At Birth

If tragedy happens and a twin dies either at birth or after, the remaining twin suffers immensely. Scripts become:

I feel there is something missing in my life (this may come to light, even if the remaining twin has not been told until years afterwards that their twin died at birth).
I did two jobs for life.
Something does not feel right.
I didn't know why I cried so much.

A puzzled look often flickers across the face and a feeling of being lost, or looking at people's faces in the street and checking—always looking for someone who isn't there.

Cord Round The Neck

Anything that jeopardises foetal life is a trauma, and a tight cord entangled round the unborn baby's body, or a tight cord round the neck, would imperil life. Imprinting scripts are:

I can't do it unless the cord somehow moves.
I'm stuck.
It's going to be a long birth—and that will annoy me.
Nobody is helping me. I am really angry.
Why don't they notice? It's too dangerous.
I'll die of strangulation.
The cord's round my neck and I'll die slowly but nobody knows and nobody cares.

Twins with cord entanglement tell their stories:

A second twin -
I feel angry.
I'm getting claustrophobic. Get off!
He's got me all knotted up.
The cord is round his neck.
Watch out for the anger. It's murderous.
He's hurting me.
A first twin -
The cords are all twisted.
He's stopping me doing anything.
Why should you get out first!
I'm first. Get out of my way.
What's he doing?
We're both trying to get out together.
Another first twin -
We're tangled up.
I'm being held back.
I can't re-enact the violence.
It's too much.
I have been born in fury with the fear of violence.

Adoption, Rage & Bullying

It is difficult to face the fact that every adopted child has suffered a devastating loss. This denial by some professionals involve with adoption causes much anger and distress with those who have been adopted, on top of the layers of anger arising out of their own primal wound of abandonment. The adopted child, with the anger of non-recognition; of not being considered; of the devastating rejection and other violent, vulnerable feelings, must not be left out of pre- and perinatal work. Here the loss and anger can be radiated and worked through, to discover a new sense of self.

Babies In A Rage

In an age where violence rages over our planet, watch baby faces carefully. A cross baby, born in anger, is telling us something. In the past, gruesome, screwed up faces and screaming voices were seen as *normal*. Sleepless nights for months on end may be the result of intra-uterine anger or cord difficulties. There may be a need for early anger imprinting to be dissipated. Feelings of betrayal are linked with anger and violence, separation and loss. Violet Oaklander in her book *Windows To Our Children* describes anger in the children she works with as being like some awful, lurking monster having to be pushed down, suppressed, deflected and avoided. Where does it come from? We believe it arises out of birth trauma.

Bullying

This is the persistent, willful, conscious desire to hurt another and put that person under stress. As bullying is aggression, then those who bully have an aggressive attitude towards parents, teachers and peers. If we connect bullying to conception, inter-uterine and birth trauma, we can see that wherever the aggressive action has come from, it is connected with fear. The child or adult who bullies may have had an aggressive reaction to a trauma near birth, with a real underlying fear of dying. Bullying may lead to many other forms of violence. So many families are in crisis because of it.

Suicide And Birth Trauma

The process of birth itself for most people may be tough, but tolerable. For others it may be devastating in its destructiveness.

Cataclysmic muscular convulsions turn, in some cases, what would have been a peaceful haven into a crushing hell.

The *no exit* phase, before the cervix begins to open, can last for hours. The sheer horror of not being able to *get out* instills thoughts of death being the answer to not feeling the pain. Intolerable pressures in later life may reinforce the suicidal thoughts.

Frank Lake wrote in 1981:

The next phase of travel through the pelvis, is at best an energetic struggle, at worst a brain destroying, suffocating, twisting, tearing, crushing torture, in which the will to live may be extinguished and a longing to die takes its place. The hazards of obstruction, impactions, prolonged delays due to uterine inertia, or sudden violent extrusion when induction puts the uterine muscle in spasm, the hazards of forceps delivery, abnormal presentations, asphyxia as a result of the cord round the neck, breech births or emergency caesarian sections, all these possibilities of profound catastrophe may occur during this phase. The will to live has often turned here into a desperate desire to die.

Working with many of these events in adult regression in the therapy room over the last twenty-five years, we believe the roots of some, if not all, types of suicide are to be found in the pre- and perinatal period. What has been produced is a lifelong imprinting of distressful feelings that have nothing to do whatever with the person's present life situations. It is a direct transcript, extraordinary, and in specific detail of the pregnant mother's disturbance, from conception to after the birth.

In the birth process, the cord round the neck could lead to hanging in later life. In one case twins were born who were not wanted. The boy was born, and nearly died at birth with the cord round the neck. At twenty-one he killed himself by hanging. Also related to the cord, is the suicidal attempt of slashing wrists, which is a typical attack on a cut bloody cord.

A scientific study carried out by Dr. Lee Salk in 1985 found that teenage suicide was related to birth trauma. They studied the obstetrical histories of a group of teenage suicides.

Out of ten perinatal risk factors, respiratory disorder, the absence of prenatal care and chronic maternal disease had the highest prevalence in suicides when compared to two matched control groups. Each of these factors occurred independently in 81% of the suicides studied.

In another study by Dr. Berti Jacobsen and Dr. Marc Bygdeman in 1987, it was found that people experiencing a painful birth were more likely to die by violent suicide in adult life. Out of a group of 645 babies born in Sweden between 1945 and 1980, 242 died by suicide by violent means between 1978 and 1995. The people who subsequently died by suicide were more likely to have been exposed to birth complications. They were therefore subjected to twice as many interventions at birth as their siblings, including forceps delivery. The researchers stipulated that obstetric procedures should be chosen to minimise pain and discomfort to the baby, because they might have a long-term effect in adulthood. They also discovered that people who asphyxiated themselves by drowning, hanging or gas inhalations were four times more likely to have suffered oxygen deprivation at birth.

Gaining insight into the pre- and perinatal period and using this knowledge is a powerful tool for understanding suicide and trying to prevent it. It provides individuals with an actual place from where their often intolerable and unbearable pain is coming.

Adults In Post Traumatic Stress Disorder (PTSD)

Trauma in the pre- and perinatal period can result in post-traumatic stress disorder in the adult, which may manifest in physical illness, injury and disease. Post-traumatic stress can be thought of as a sane reaction to an insane situation. When a person experiences strong reactions to ugly and abusive events in life it does not mean they are crazy.

Doctors with expertise in trauma have noted that in order to survive any normal human being—whatever that means—when placed in extremely demanding circumstances will develop exceptional ways of mentally coping with the situation. Many of the symptoms of post-traumatic stress disorder, in war veterans and other trauma survivors are in fact ways of acting, thinking, feeling and moving that were originally developed to promote the possibility of survival in exceptional situations. These adults live much of their lives in combat mode, which becomes their mode of survival in the war zones of life.

It has been observed that some war veterans do not suffer any effects of PTSD while others are debilitated from it. If fractal patterns are to be believed, my hypothesis is that those soldiers who suffered trauma and damage in the pre and perinatal period would be more susceptible to PTSD. When faced with the trauma of war, they would be more likely to suffer personality changes, the appearance of personality disorders and Gulf War Syndrome, than those whose life in the womb and childhood were less traumatic. In both cases, it may be the effects that are life-destroying at the extreme end.

When working with clients throughout the spectrum of humanistic and integrative psychotherapy, I believe an individual has to recognise and be ready to say:

"There are reactions that sometimes go on inside of me—in my thoughts in my feelings in my ways of acting, in my body, that have something to do with combat reflexes. These are reactions to situations happening now with a way of acting that is meant to be used in survival situations, even when what is happening now isn't a question of survival but it feels like it."

Symptoms Of Post-Traumatic Stress Disorder

1.   *Vigilance and scanning: constant checking of what is happening around.*
2.   *Elevated startle response: being jumpy when something surprising happens.*
3.   *Blunted affect or psychic numbing: a reduction or loss of the ability to feel.*
4.   *Aggressive controlling behaviour : acting with violence; using force to get your own way.*
5.   *Interruption of memory and concentration: excellent at times and then severely interrupted by exposure to an experience which causes a stress reaction.*
6.   *Depression: exhaustion, negative attitude, apathy.*
7.   *General anxiety: body tension, back cramps, stomach cramps, headaches, paranoid fears.*
8.   *Sustained feelings of fear and guilt.*
9.   *Episodes of anger and rage.*
10. *Substance abuse: drugs, alcohol, etc.*
11. *Dissociative experiences: a person behaves as though they were back in the type of situation they faced during the trauma.*
12. *Insomnia: difficulty in sleeping.*
13. *Suicidal feelings and ideas.*
14. *Survivor guilt: when others do not survive.*

Health Problems Arising Out Of Birth Trauma

All the factors mentioned above may be applied to trauma in the pre- and perinatal period but I want to specifically apply this to injury, disease and illness manifesting in the adult from this period of life.

Some of these injuries and health problems may be due to the ill health of the mother during the pregnancy and at the time of birth affected by her emotional mental state. From the disciplines of pre- and perinatal psychotherapy and pre- and perinatal psychology, have come the findings that trauma and abuse—both internally and externally, either intentionally or by accident during pregnancy—can seriously damage the foetus in utero.

There are also worldwide prolific findings of traumatic births causing brain damage, injuries to eyes and eyesight, maladjusted behaviour, possible dyslexia, learning difficulties, violent behaviour and bullying—to name but a few.

Some of these illnesses may be due to damage to the foetus by lack of oxygen; placental deficiency; the foetus getting tied up in its umbilical cord; the foetus being marinated in mothers illness; the struggle of the foetus to survive physical battering of the mother, or the consumption of alcohol drugs and other substance abuse. At birth possible brain damage, spinal cord limb and organ damage may be the reason—the list is endless.

Breathing Problems

One young man came to me when his mother was dying of multiple sclerosis. His major presenting symptoms were that he could not move from his job, his home or his parents. He had a panic reaction every time movement was suggested. He had no personal identity and was lost in his mother's trauma of illness. He had recurring asthma, panicked every time and then could not breathe. He was in a permanent state of shock and jumped markedly at the slightest sound. Regressing to his intra-uterine life and birth trauma, he found that he had been marinated in his mother's sickness and was born in shock. Owing to breathing difficulties at birth, he had a tracheotomy.

This surgical, operation was a terrible birth trauma. He had lived permanently in this state of post-traumatic stress until he discovered the traumas that were blocking him. He was only intermittently out of the shock for some years but has made great strides and changes to better life. His breathing problems are much improved and the quality of his own life style changed beyond recognition.

Pelvic Pain

Richard came to us suffering from chronic, intense pain in the right hip. The pain had persisted and intensified in recent months. He visited numerous conventional medical practitioners specialists in their chosen field. The diagnoses ranged from *an anteriorly displaced fifth lumbar vertebrae* to *ankylosing of the sacroiliac joint*. He reluctantly took charge for a while and declined the offer of surgery—to this day he does not know which part of his body was to be removed. He came to Amethyst to explore his pre-birth memories with us. This was his story:

During regression, I experienced in the womb prolonged periods of inactivity; feeling hopelessly stuck and trapped. I also suffered acute physical pain due to concentrated and intense pressure on my right hip. I was unable to struggle free from this discomfort because I was so badly tied up with the umbilical cord. It was too much to tolerate and integrate at the time. The primal pain became locked into my sub-conscious, only to surface later in my life at a time of great stress, when my wife and I separated. Having visited Amethyst on six occasions during the last eighteen months, this experience has changed my life. I am now almost free of back pain and the abdominal cramps which plagued me for so long. My sleeping patterns have improved and I feel I am a much content and relaxed personality both in myself and in my relationship with others.

Damage To The Immune System

Our thoughts also influence the chemical balance of the immune system. Under prolonged stress we are more likely to be susceptible to a variety of diseases, including cancer, infectious diseases, auto immune disease and allergies. All these can affect the foetus in the womb.

People develop specific immune system reactions to defend the body from being overwhelmed by particular kinds of germs. So too can people develop specific reactions to defend the mind against being overwhelmed by particular memories.

It is a natural and healthy action of the human mind in such circumstances to take steps to ease the discomfort.

Trauma In The Psyche

It is believed that the human organism has the ability to heal itself naturally but I believe it also needs help. When trauma has gone deep into the psyche sometimes it is necessary for the therapist to help the clients return to the trauma at the same amplitude or frequency when the original trauma occurred. Layers may be uncovered but the depth to which the clients go must be determined by the client themselves.

Cancer And Post Traumatic Stress Disorder In Utero

We are told that we were all born with cancer cells in our bodies. The cancerous cell is a low-frequency, low-amplitude embryonic cell. This means that the cell, instead of vibrating at the same rate of the body, vibrates at a much slower energy or frequency—the same frequency as that of embryonic cells. When a cell slows its vibration, the body thinks it is making a baby and subsequently allows the cell to multiply and divide rapidly, which is what causes a tumerous growth. Then it sends in blood supply to feed those cells; most tumours, if they are not treated grow at the same rate that a baby grows.

In the first trimester of life these cells are developing at this speed. If a trauma occurs to the mother at this time when she may or may not be aware that she is pregnant, the foetus becomes marinated in the trauma. In adult life if a situation triggers a similar traumatic situation to that which occurred in the foetus, do cancer cells begin to develop in the first trimester of life and is cancer a post traumatic stress disorder manifesting as disease from early prenatal trauma? This can be applied to many more diseases that may have their origins in utero.

Stress is said to be the cause of many illnesses in the developing child and adult, so it follows that post-traumatic stress disorder resulting from trauma in the womb or at birth may be the cause of illness and disease. I believe many people are completely unaware how far back some of their illnesses go and how their health is affected by post traumatic stress disorder resulting from trauma in the pre- and perinatal period.

Chapter 6

BIRTH TRAUMA IN BABIES AND CHILDREN

Birth Trauma In Babies And Children

Some years ago I received a phone call from the Gerry Ryan Show, on Irish National Radio, as they are aware of the pre- and perinatal therapeutic work we do at Amethyst with adults and children. A distressed mother phoned in for help as her fourteen month old son screamed and cried in his sleep relentlessly and the family had not had a good night's sleep since he was born. Her concern was for her son and what could be causing his distress. I spoke to her on the programme, and recognising the symptoms were probably related to birth trauma, I asked her what her son's birth had been like. She responded that she was in hospital, she had been awake but he had the cord round his neck which had caused him, and her, great distress.

I simply suggested that this was a possible birth trauma and there was a treatment developed by William Emerson called Birth Simulating Massage to treat infant birth trauma. It was something that she could do herself for her baby and involved gentle stroking and holding patterns, simulating pressures on the infant's body that were most traumatised during birth.

As this sounded like a cord trauma I suggested that she held her baby and loved him, talked gently to him and then very gently stroked and massaged his neck briefly. His reaction would probably be to scream and cry if the distress was coming from the trauma of the cord round his neck, so it was very important to affirm and love him in between the stroking and massaging. This treatment would help to desensitise the trauma that was still possibly causing his distress.

Twenty four hours later she phoned me—it had worked—they had all had the best night's sleep in fourteen months! Her son had reacted by screaming and crying as she intuitively stroked his neck. A week later she phoned again. The treatment had dramatically dissipated the symptoms, all was now peaceful and her baby son was no longer distressed.

Time and time again we have feedback from parents when it has been suggested that some of their children's problems may be stemming from birth trauma. Much of it is positive.

I remember over thirty years ago as a teacher I was very involved in teaching the children with behavioural, emotional and learning difficulties.

Some mothers would comment that their child had a difficult birth and they were sure it had affected their son or daughter. How right they were, but it wasn't until I met Dr. Frank Lake in the 1970's that I had any idea of the research and experiential work that was going on with adults, which was later to help infants and children. All of this research and development except for a minimum of exploratory investigation was directed towards adult patients.

Birth Psychology

In the mid 1970's and early 1980's it was time for the children to be considered—if birth trauma affects adults, what are the odds that children are also affected and need help. A great deal of research has gone into finding evidence for the full range of infant capabilities, whether from personal reports contributed by parents, revelations arising from therapeutic work or from formal experiments.

Amongst the most outstanding researchers are Thomas Verny and the late David Chamberlain, both pioneers in birth psychology. They founded the Pre and Perinatal Psychology Association of North America (PPPANA) in 1983. It is now renamed The Association for Pre and Perinatal Psychology and Health (APPPAH).

They and members of the Association are continuing to research the impacts of pre and perinatal experiences worldwide. In 1981 Thomas Verny, the Canadian psychiatrist published his best selling book *The Secret Life of the Unborn Child* and in it he wrote:-

There is a growing body of empirical studies showing significant relationships between birth trauma and a number of specific difficulties; violence, criminal behaviour, learning disabilities, epilepsy, hyperactivity and child alcohol and drug abuse.

In 1988 David Chamberlain, an American psychologist practising in San Diego, California, published his groundbreaking book *Babies Remember Birth*. Also translated into many languages it has now been reprinted under the title *The Mind of your Newborn Baby.*

The leading researcher in the world for treatment with birth traumatised infants and children is Californian psychologist and psychotherapist, Dr. William Emerson. He began the development and research for infants and children in 1974. In the autumn of 1976 he visited Frank Lake in England in order to study birth and prenatal phenomena with him.

Emerson began to question whether infants and children would benefit from forms of treatment especially developed for them.To try and evaluate this, Emerson conducted a series of parent-child workshops throughout Europe in the late 1970's and early 1980's with children ranging from three to thirteen.

His main focus was to clarify ordinary or unusual difficulties the children were having, and to experimentally use birth discussions, music and birth games to ascertain possible traumatic antecedents. He wrote in 1984:

"Birth issues were rampant in the art, fantasies and dreams of the children, especially before the age of eight. Birth and play were temperamentally related; the moodier the child, the more severe the difficulties the children were having, the more intense and frequent were birth issues. Ninety five percent of the children were able to remember significant aspects presenting difficulties."

Treatment Of An Infant

In one case, William treated a traumatised infant with asthma, using his Birth Simulating Massage. To simulate pressures of the uterus and pelvis during birth, gentle massage is applied to the affected areas where there has been pressure on the infant's body during the birth process. These places can be automatically and spontaneously found as the baby reacts to certain areas that are massaged. The emotional work is largely complete when there is no emotional reaction to the simulated birth pressure.

In this infant, the symptoms were dramatically altered after two one-hour sessions and completely resolved after three. Asthmatic children are prone to a high incidence of bronchial, lung, ear, nose and throat symptoms. A fifteen-year follow up of this child reported no further bronchial or asthmatic episodes, and very low incidents of coughs or colds.

As their emotional work is complete, another phase begins which Emerson calls schematic repatterning. His thoughts are that the movement patterns that babies use to get from the uterus to the outside world are deeply imbedded and retained in the nervous system and body. These movement patterns he calls *birth schema*, which may be referred to by others as *life scripts*, *colouring of life patterns*, *learned responses* or *behaviour traits;* they may be positive or dysfunctional in their impacts. The action patterns or response learned behaviour from traumatic births do change as these trauma dissipate during treatment.

Recognising Birth Trauma Related Problems

Parents bring children into treatment for birth trauma when they know their child had a difficult birth and when there may be disturbed behaviour relating to it—although until it is brought to their attention the parents may not have the knowledge that the two events may be related.

When parents hear that babies remember birth they may feel guilty —but there is no need for parental guilt. Often it is not the type of birth they themselves would have wanted for their baby. Sometimes they are caught up in the type of birth prevalent at the time. No mother or father wants a stressful pregnancy or traumatic birth but it can result from a number of factors like relationship difficulties, environmental problems, unemployment, ill-health—all of which contribute to the pressures of life.

Medical classifications for birth trauma are breech, forceps, vacuum extraction, caesarian delivery and anaesthesia. From our research we would also add induction, premature birth and also late arrival.

The type of behaviour parents may observe in their children related to birth trauma may be:-

aggression, excessive anger, anxiety, nervousness, not relating to other siblings or parents, insecurity, hanging on or excessive pleasing, stuck in fears like sleeping in the dark, excessive screaming or crying, not eating well, weight loss, separation anxieties at being left at school.

Hyperactive children also need positive help:

Tom was a hyperactive child and had a most erratic sleep pattern. His mother continued a very busy teaching job during the pregnancy—hardly having time for his birth before she went back to work. Tom's hyperactivity in the family with siblings was almost impossible. When he was seven he was given a violin and at the age of ten was able to play five different musical instruments. Twenty years later he is a successful professional solo violinist.

Hyperactive children are usually very creative and there are ways to channel the energy. When I was ten my own father gave me a hockey stick—which eventually channelled my energy into becoming a professional sportswoman!

The withdrawn child may need to retreat from a world which is too painful. The quiet or shy child may not be brought for help. They are often seen as *good* by parents, being well-behaved and not troublesome. Violet Oaklander pointed out in 1978 that the problem only becomes evident when the shy behaviour is exaggerated through the child hardly ever speaking, or whispering. They may become '*loners*', have few friends and become the object of bullying.

Birth-Related Difficulties

Each of our births is different which may in part be the reason why each of us is unique. There are many other birth issues but the following are brief and general guidelines.

• *Early or premature babies* may want to arrive early for everything and be anxious not to be late—but they may never feel ready for anything. They may react as though there is not enough time and may feel rushed by others, causing an irrational aggression. Parents may have difficulties if they try to push their children too soon to do things—the child may want to stand on the sidelines and watch.

• *Late or postmaturity babies* may not want to take the initiative. They may get very anxious if they are late but will probably feel they are running out of time—but still leave things until the very last minute! It may take *'late'* babies a long time to get going and may perhaps be late developers and slow in learning. The greater frustration may be with the parents!

• *Caesarian babies* may sit back and wait for everything to be done for them. They lack self empowerment and self worth—being *'taken out'* they did not have the vaginal struggle and feel they haven't done anything to deserve what they have. The parents of caesarian borns have the difficult task of teaching their children how to do things for themselves, and to teach them boundaries that they never had like vaginal borns. They will probably do the opposite to what you say! And help is seen as a put down or a disempowerment. There is also the possibility that parents may not be able to get them out of the house as they grow older—and they may need some physical assistance!

• *Anaesthetised babies* may blame parents for their inability to function. They may have difficulty taking responsibility for their own actions. When trying to relate with them you may experience a *fading in and out*. They may have low energy, deaden their feelings and their contact and are often difficult to *reach*. Their concentration can be seriously affected. There is an added observation from research that *anaethetised* children as they get older may turn to drugs to *escape from the pressures of life*. Another reason for turning to drugs may be to avoid pain—as their mothers did during labour.

*   ***Babies are induced*** due to lack of progression, eg contract—ions are not strong enough; mother is ill; when labour needs to be started for external reasons. Induced children are usually

    very stubborn. They have problems getting started and will resent being told what to do; *"Wait—I'm not doing this until I am ready—then I'll do it my way."* They may not see another person's point of view, may be quite contrary and say "No" to any suggestion.

*   ***Breech-born*** babies are either born buttocks or feet first—it is a violent birth and the baby often becomes a victim. They cannot get things in order and others will wonder why they can't do things which seem quite natural to them. They will keep trying but seem to get nothing right. They may well be in conflict with themselves and parents and display disappointment to self and others. There is a tendency to passive anger and an inner violence.

*   ***Babies need forceps*** because they are stuck and cannot get out fast enough. It may be due to a large head, mother's small pelvis, insufficient contractions and a complicated presentation. The birth is violent—help comes at last but can that support ever be trusted again? They will start something but have difficulty finishing it because of all the obstructions or distractions on the way. They may appear as being cut off from their emotions and be shy and withdrawn, and be prone to headaches and nausea. It is quite remarkable in a traumatic forceps birth which has developed into a body schema, that the child will reach a point of confusion in conversation. At this point the head shakes back and forth as the child is trying to wrestle free of the forceps and the current argument, his or her forceps/oppositional personality has got him or her into!

Bullying

Bullying is a behavioural problem affecting the lives of thousands of school children and their families. At primary school level over one in ten children are involved in bullying on a frequent basis. Research carried out by Dr. Mora O'Moore in 1994 found that one child in five is afraid to go to school because of the fear of being bullied.

Bullying is the persistant, willful, conscious desire to hurt another and put that person under stress. It is carried out through verbal, physical, gesture, exclusion and extortion bullying.

As bullying is aggression then children who bully have an aggressive attitude towards peers, parents and teachers. Connecting bullying to birth trauma, all aggressive actions come from fear. The child who bullies may have had an aggressive reaction to a traumatic birth with a real underlying fear of dying. If bullying is intentional to hurt others, it is possible that the bullying related to birth trauma might be unconscious revenge on the forceps.

The child that is bullied may have a passive reaction to a traumatic birth with a real fear of dying. The victim is often seen as different, he/she may be hypersensitive, cautious, anxious, passive or submissive and are not determined, forceful or decisive. A report published by the charity Kidscape in 1998 found that children who were bullied at school are up to seven times more likely to try to kill themselves. More research is needed—even by schools to note down on children's record cards the type of birth they had and whether there is any correlation to behaviour patterns later.

A leading question is whether the type of birth trauma a child has experienced leads to bullying, and also to types of suicide attempts. Research evidence shows for example that the cord round the neck may lead to suicide by hanging; a drugged birth may lead to overdose; and gas or anaesthetic at birth may lead to death by car exhaust fumes that used to be the gas oven asphyxiation.

Chapter 7

WORK AT AMETHYST

Work At Amethyst With Infants, Children And Teenagers

Carmel Byrne and I have worked with infants, children and teenagers—and also teach parents, therapists and others the different techniques for birth trauma healing. They include play therapy, storytelling as in birth stories, animal stories to reach aggression, birth simulating massage, movement and mime, painting, art, toys, role play, sand trays, birth games, tents, caterpillar tunnels and cushions. The improvisation and restructuring of birth trauma with babies from six weeks old is done using gentle massage and music with energy healing work.

Carmel Byrne stresses that although children go into traumatised states it is done by play therapy, gently and in small groups. The parents are present if possible with other family members, brothers, sisters, grandparents who may be instrumental to the success of the empathic process. There is immediate bonding with loving cuddles with Mummy and Daddy, often with soft music in the background.

Working With Induction And Breech Birth Trauma

A distraught mother brought Michael, her eleven year old son, to Carmel. The major problems were his fear of the dark, he was dyslexic and was never ready for anything whether he liked where he was going or not. Getting him ready for a party or school was impossible—he would play with the dog, his toys, his computer games or read a book.

The mother knew his birth had been difficult—and the baby was not ready to be born. The hospital said he was so the delivery was induced and he was born breech. The therapist prepared the room with toys, a child's tent and a caterpillar tunnel to be used to simulate the womb experience. The toy he chose was a large, brown, lanky monkey which could pass as the placenta—Michael said it was his monster.

He did understand he was reliving his birth. The room was darkened gradually by drawing the curtains and Michael played in his tent. He came out of the tent feet first, always stating he was not ready and it wasn't the right way. This was helping him desensitise his breech birth and letting him do it in his own time

In the sixth session he stated that however long it took he would do it his way. So he went into his tent and sat and sat. Suddenly he said,

"I'm ready now", "Is there anybody there at all?"

There was silence as the therapist and mother listened to him.

"Listen to me," he shouted and got into a terrible rage.

Cushions were put at the end of the tunnel and Michael came out head first, doing it his way and empowering himself. No more sessions were needed and mother reported that Michael was studying better at school, he was no longer afraid of the dark and the constant struggle of not being on time had dissipated.

Energy Healing

Babies and children are very responsive to the use of energy healing within a play or therapy session.

A single mother brought along her seven month old baby Katy to Carmel because she had a hole in the heart that had developed at seven months in utero. The mother knew that Katy's birth had been difficult with a long labour. Birth was a high forceps delivery, the baby was born purple with distress, was choking and had difficulty breathing. She was thought to be dying, was resuscitated and put into intensive care.

During the second session of healing Katy turned purple, went very cold and her breathing became erratic. Her mother remarked that this was how her birth had been. As Carmel Byrne held Katy's head very gently, it became a birth trauma session involving gentle stroking to desensitise the trauma of the forceps. The mother continued to bring Katy for healing for well over a year. At sixteen months of age Katy went for her medical check up and the hole in the heart was smaller. By the time Katy was eighteen months of age, the hole in the heart had closed.

Healing Severe Birth Trauma

Colette, a baby aged eighteen months, was brought by her parents to Carmel because she was crying excessively, was not sleeping day or night, and screamed in terror and rage if she was touched, particularly on the head. Her father stressed that her screams at night were terrifying.

Colette had two previous sessions in which she experienced severe birth trauma and screamed in rage and terror. After the first session there was a distinct improvement, she could be pacified and touched but still was not sleeping. Before the second session, on talking with the mother, Carmel discovered the mother's sleep pattern when carrying Colette had been one of studying night and day for her external exams. They both agreed that this could have set up Colette's own disturbed sleep patterns.

After the second session in which she explored a little more birth trauma, the crying ceased and Colette was able to stay quiet and play with her toys in the cot.

She was brought back for a third session into the Amethyst training group for review with her three year old brother Timmy. There had been considerable improvement and she was much better at allowing people to touch her. The group were shown how to develop a session playing with toys, to help the child get used to strangers, how to play birth games, for example, crawling through daddy's legs to restimulate the birth trauma and desensitise it. The children got great affirmation from the group.

The major game for the session was the earthquake game where Colette was placed between mummy and daddy as they sat closely facing each other on the floor, with their arms around each other. Earthquake music or womb sounds were played and the children made their own sounds.

Colette it was discovered, was to do it in her own way in this session. She automatically went into her birth process. She made an attempt at getting out but went back. She stayed contentedly and tried again quietly but retreated again. In her birth she had her head engaged for a long time. When the head started crowning, Carmel gently placed her hands on Colette's head, with Timmy helping. Carmel affirmed Colette all the time—

"Good girl, do it your way", whilst her hands were gently massaging Colette's head. At this point her head was engaged, her nose was squashed—so no pressure was applied. Her head appeared, with distressed crying, and one little hand popped out. The *'hole'* for her to appear from was beneath her parent's locked arms. Colette was eased out gently by Carmel, helped by Timmy, and handed immediately to mummy and daddy for instant bonding. The recovery time was rapid and mummy and daddy made a human boat for the children to sit in whilst quiet music was played. After this session the parents said that Colette was, *"A new child."*

There Is Some Hope

The adults who witnessed Colette experiencing her birth were very moved by it. One member put it succinctly:-

All I could think of was how privileged Timmy and Colette were. I was looking at Colette and she was so happy and content at being in the womb. She had her mother and father there, as she was coming out, and she could have come out at any time—but there was a residue of her birth. Once she got out, there was this cocoon in the womb of family relationships that she could actually go into.

It may seem horrific putting a baby through this, especially when you see the pain they go through. But the healing is saving them from a lifetime of pain. It may be far better to treat birth related trauma in the early years, through the many techniques that are now available, to prevent dysfunctional behaviour emerging in later years from unresolved traumatisation.

Chapter 8

TRAUMATIC INTRA-UTERINE EVENTS

Drawing on our experiences at Amethyst, we will now explore the time before birth, reaching back as far as conception.

Frank Lake Explores Intra-Uterine Life

According to Frank Lake, some participants in his primaling seminars would have a clear idea of what undisturbed intra-uterine life is like. It is a good place and there the foetus is *God, at the very centre of things*. The foetus would *shimmer with ecstatic feeling*. However, other participants would have a realistic recollection of a bad womb experience. These negative intra—uterine experiences are the focus of this chapter, and they include foetal crises, diseases, emotional upheavals in the mother, a twin situation, and attempted abortion.

For Lake, all this research was done experientially, in a therapeutic situation, by re-birthing adults, whose present life was blocked emotionally, causing behaviour disturbances and relation—ship difficulties. He points out that if each positive stage of growth is not properly facilitated, an incomplete phase contaminates the next phase and therefore past-contaminated transitions contaminate present ones. In other words the character, behaviour and emotional disturbances worsen and the individual may become labelled as maladjusted, unteachable, delinquent or unmanageable.

As a result of his research, towards the end of his life Lake concluded that the origin of every trauma does not after all lie in birth, but rather in the experiences of a foetus during its first three months, beginning with conception. How parents react when they find out they are expecting a child is the first impacting experience. This means that early trauma of the first days and weeks repeats itself during the rest of the pregnancy, becomes a pattern in birth, and continues into infancy and childhood.

Foetal Crises

So much of the distress in the womb from external events causes severe pain in the foetus.

Blunt Trauma: accidents, falls, assault, a near death experience for baby, may trigger premature delivery. External abuse is experienced by the foetus and is a tragic, horrific reliving by an adult in regression.

The helpless foetus is marinated in the external anger and rage of the perpetrator and the responses of mother to be. Scripts are:

He's hitting my mother.
I'm inside and I can feel him hitting her. I'm raging.
He still has the power to hurt me.

This type of event may lead to countless examples of anger and terror in adult behaviour.

Drug Taking In Mother: Suicide attempts by an overdose of drugs by an adult may be related to drugs taken by mother during the pregnancy, or linked to anaesthesia during the birth process.

Tobacco Smoking: Smoking provokes real anger in the unborn, Mothers who smoke will send their babies into respiratory distress. Elizabeth Noble in her 1993 book *Primal Connections* observed this with the use of ultrasound. In regression, the foetus feels real anger. The scripts are:

Stop smoking—you are killing me.
My brain is splitting. It's split down the middle. The smell is smoky.
I'm not going to let you make me sick.

A 1992 research paper by Irving, Neto and Vemy has shown that there is a significant relationship between drugs, maternal stress and anger. In one study it was found that a fear of losing one's temper was more often reported by those whose mothers smoked cigarettes (30%) than those whose mothers did not smoke (24%) during pregnancy. A fear of becoming violent and destructive was more often reported by those whose mothers used cigarettes (25%) marijuana (44%) or alcohol (34%) than by those whose mothers did not use these agents.

A Mother's Feelings Of Grief

Frank Lake told the story of a Swedish architect who came to a workshop.

This was a man with a lot of colour in his life. He deliberately put colour into his life, but deep down he felt a bitter sadness and angry resentment. This was foreign to him, but yet also too familiar. It invaded him in a way he could not prevent. This imprinted his life with a greyness he did not want. He felt he was where he did not want to be, but this was nonsense, because he was. When he experienced the regression visualisation back to conception, he realised that his sense of inner greyness came from his mother. Two years before his birth, she had been forced to leave her homeland and flee, leaving everything behind her. This caused her great sadness and angry resentment, which he picked up when he was in the womb. These were his mother's feelings and did not belong to him. As he returned them to her in his therapy session the greyness left him. He had chosen to be an architect in order to bring light and colour into life.

A Lack Of Bonding

A lack of bonding throughout pregnancy is a major component of dysfunction.

One client had no recognition in the womb by mother who didn't realise she was pregnant but was delighted when she discovered her pregnancy at six months. This child grew up with excessive attention seeking. As a university lecturer he was always in the limelight but this was never enough. He was in danger of wrecking his relationship with his wife. On re-experiencing this time in the womb, he encountered a colossal rage with his mother for the non-recognition. This anger was ruining his relationships until he discovered where it came from. His life and relationships improved because he learned to change his inappropriate behaviour.

Sexual Intercourse/Rape

Time and again the foetus experiences the occasions when the parents are making love. Real feelings, of sometimes misinterpreted, physical and mental abuse can be experienced, but when the lovemaking is violent the foetus is aware and attitudes to sex can well be formed in this situation.

We had often associated sexual problems with the umbilical cord and the feelings coming through, but there seems to be yet another way of communicating these feelings, as if they are marinated right through the cells.

An extraordinary number of clients experienced the sperm being ejaculated, and felt dirty, sticky, frightened and were also aware of mother's feelings to the act of lovemaking. The number of clients experiencing this as sexual abuse raises the question of how love-making is approached during pregnancy.

The Wrong Gender

To experience being a boy when a girl was wanted is a pretty painful event. And the foetus often is aware in the womb that they are not the gender the parents want. To be a boy when there have been one, two, three, four and even five boys before you arrive—it is a wonder that anything has ever gone right in your life. Scripts are:

I always get it wrong.
I am such a disappointment. I can't please anyone.
I want you to love me. I'll die without love. She doesn't want me.
I'm in a double bind—she wants me but I'm all wrong.

Amniocentesis

The medical doctor inserted a needle into the client's mother's cervix when she thought she was pregnant. It is the process of amniocentesis, where amniotic fluid is withdrawn from the pregnant mother with a hollow needle poked through the belly or cervix. If abortion is not considered a real possibility, or genetic defects, amniocentesis has no purpose. It is highly dangerous to the developing baby, as accidents do occur, damaging the foetus. What the professional pushing the diagnostic tool does not know is the possibility of permanent damage such a procedure may cause. The foetus, in baby logic, may interpret this as attempted murder, and may also confuse it with attempted abortion. If there is any bonding at all the *'accident'* will cause permanent cutting of the bonding and mother and child may be estranged for life. Survivors of attempted abortion suffer serious consequences. The trauma is overwhelming, leaving the person changed and disconnected from their bodies.

Chamberlain wrote in 1998 that now amniocentesis is common, babies in the womb frequently confront a needle entering their private domain. Ultrasound studies show that babies react fearfully, defensively and sometimes aggressively. Chamberlain relates a story of a pregnant woman's experience during amniocentesis.

Her husband, the doctor and the ultrasound technician all saw little unborn Claire bat the needle. The technician said, "Take it out!" When the doctor reinserted the needle, the foetus again attacked it, forcing the doctor to remove the needle. The husband and doctor were in a nervous sweat.

The doctor said he had never seen a baby bat a needle before. Who wouldn't be angry at this intrusion!

Much of the violence which takes place in utero is the silent invisible type; Chamberlain wrote in 1998 that the injuries cannot be discovered until much later. Babies are trying to alert us to this damage but we are slow in learning. It is often stated that silent, passive anger is the killer. Anger may be a protection to the truth, it may disempower —until it finds its roots and the truth and empowerment are realised. Scripts of hidden anger are:

Anger covers up pain, despair and sadness. It shouldn't be like this.
I can't get angry with people or tell them how they affect me.

Diseases

Serious illness to the mother often resulted in the child being in shock for most if not all of its life. Scripts are:

I am sick. It's my fault she's sick. I feel dragged down.
If I make a big effort to get what I want, it won't be what I want.
This amount of closeness makes me sick.
I wasn't able to be fed—milk made me sick.
Must be something wrong with me.
Always expecting something and getting nothing back. It's all my fault.

Sadly, a person can be sick for most of their life and never understand why. It can be mother's illness they are carrying in memory form. It is vital for the client to separate out his or her own feelings from mother's from these early periods for healing to take place.

A Sick Mother

Mary's mother was sick with tuberculosis when Mary was conceived, was in utero and when she was born. Mary throughout life had a multitude of problems and lived in a non-feeling, frightening world. She was depressed from birth with intrusive recall and dissociative experiences. In therapy Mary felt she had been poisoned, not only by mother's illness but also by mother's constant smoking. She felt dirty, rejected and no good. This manifested in not only emotional and mental problems but severe premenstrual tension, which today is being alleviated by a gradual reliving and realisation of what life in the womb was like for her.

Emotional Upheavals For The Mother

We have seen how the invasion of the foetus by maternal distress, from the mother's often complex emotions, is experienced by what Lake called the Maternal Foetal Distress Syndrome and Mott called Negative Umbilical Affect. This denotes the feeling state of the foetus as brought about by blood circulating through the umbilical cord from the mother.

There are now many scientific research studies producing possible evidence as to why this happens, e.g. Candace Pert and her studies of neuropeptides and their receptors as the biochemical correlates of emotions. The suffering foetus states,

I'm in a dreadful place. I can't stand it.

And so, the suicidal tendencies are sown.

Continuing Lake's research, we have confirmed that the umbilicus is the predominant mechanism by which the positive or negative feelings of the mother from her life situations and her personal reactions to them, are transmitted to the foetus. So when mother is angry or terrified any time throughout the nine months of her pregnancy, the unborn baby is invaded by these feelings and every cell of the unborn is marinated and informed of the emotional crisis.

The unborn's own emotions and reactions to the crisis are present. This does appear to be the source of many of the adverse, angry feelings felt by us in later life, whether as children or adults.

Mother's Negative Reaction To The Pregnancy

This research makes clear that Mother's reaction to her pregnancy can have a great effect on the new human organism. Total lack of recognition leads the foetus to feel degraded, unwanted and rejected. The terror is a direct result of what Frank calls transmarginal stress in the foetus. The revulsion turns inwards and becomes a profound and permanent sense of worthlessness. The scripts can be:

No one wants me. No one loves me.

I've got it wrong. I'm never right. I'm no good.

I wish I weren't here.

I'm insignificant. I want some recognition. It's my fault. I feel guilty.

The Effects Of Foetal Affliction

Our experience of spending thousands of hours with those reliving the effects of maternal foetal distress gives us significant evidence, as Lake before had found, that affliction can activate a mechanism causing a *murderous splitting*.

The foetal victim displaces the anger and other emotions throughout the body in a severe overwhelming fashion. This displacement, localisation and disposal of negative umbilical affect appears to give rise to mental anguish in the roots of the schizoid, paranoid and hysterical personality disorders.

When anger, rage and violence are displaced into the unborn baby's body, physical ailments appear in the child, teenager or adult in later life. It seems a possible cause for the roots of many diseases and psychosomatic illnesses as the inturned anger destroys the cells of the body. Where the anger has never been able to be expressed by the client it results in inner destruction and illness. Some examples of displaced anger are:-

In the head — migraine, bad heads
In the eyes — looking daggers, looks can kill
In the jaw — clenched jaw, oral tension
In the lungs — coughing, choking, breathlessness
Asthma — the cry of rage
Fear of cancer — what is inside me will kill me

The link between depression in the adult and frozen anger derived from womb trauma is evident from our work. There may be a strong link between some forms of lifetime depression and the silent, inexpressible anger from the womb—as the blocked and retroflected rage is having to take in so much badness along with the good. The pain feeds the rage.

Tragedies In The Wider World

Tragedies in the wider world can cause distress to both mother and child. Lake himself often quoted an experience he had in Chicago when he was lecturing on the maternal foetal distress syndrome. Afterwards a mother came excitedly to him saying what he had said explained for the first time the behaviour of one of her daughters.

Apparently her daughter and other members of her class kept bursting into tears for no obvious reason. They did not know why. At Frank Lake's lecture she realised that they had all been in the womb when JFK was assassinated, which sent shock waves and grief throughout the whole nation. It didn't solve anything but maybe healed something by giving a reason for behaviour that was completely unexplainable before.

Attempted Abortion

The rejected foetus suffers, but never so deeply as the survivors of attempted abortion. They are deeply aware of annihilation, rejection and the risk of being *wiped out*. This sense of not being wanted permeates all areas of life and the desire to end it all is great. In regression the adult reliving the feelings of this suffering foetus knows its life is in danger and relives his or her near-murder with quite shocking accuracy and overwhelming terror. Attempted abortion scripts, like those of the adopted baby, are of complete rejection:

I am a mistake. I shouldn't be here.
I have to block pain—it hurts so.
I feel so tense all the time.
I don't know if I am wanted or not.
I can't forget—but I can't do anything about it.
I am going to split wide open.
I'm going to die—I'm going to hell.

The implications for survivors of attempted abortion or near spontaneous abortion, including near accidental miscarriage, is horrifically stressful. The foetus, as we have learned from the reliving of attempted and failed abortions, knows its presence is resented and its life is in danger.

It relives its own near murder, terror of death, with quite astounding accuracy. The enormous feelings of rejection and the murderous rage surrounding its own near annihilation throughout adult life are a serious and misunderstood affliction for many who have survived this horror.

An Abortion Attempt Discovered - A Client Speaks Out

I was in the womb. I was very, very tiny. I could feel my head. The pain in my head was ferocious. Something was there with me in this black hole. It was threatening me. I wanted to connect with my mother but she just wasn't there. It felt like she was dead. I so wanted to connect but there was no response. I was alive but in a dead womb. Nothing or no-one cared or was there to look after me.

I felt a hard point, thin and sharp prod me. The terror filled every cell of me. I felt the point, thin and hard, prod my spine and travel to my brain. My brain felt as though it were exploding. My head was bursting with pain. Then I went completely numb. The feeling was the same as I get as an adult—the silent scream, the loss of words in an overwhelming situation. The split and the autism, when I can't find the words in a social setting I just dissociate.

I bonded to rejection—there was nothing else to bond with. The feelings of terror, isolation and abandonment were so overwhelming. The fear of falling into that black hole was very real—like falling into a bottomless pit. It was like falling into the abyss of not belonging and non-being. I felt so cut off. I was also aware of my twin sister, and possibly a brother too. She was beside me, she was alive. Suddenly in a blinding flash she disappeared, she'd gone. I was in a treble trauma—I almost lost my own life with that needle; if there was ever any contact or bonding with my mother had disappeared and was non-existent and my twin sister was lost to me. There had been a deep bond between us and I thought I could not live without her.

As can be seen from this story, the implications for survivors of attempted abortion or near spontaneous abortion, including near accidental miscarriage, are deeply distressing. The foetus, as we have learned from the reliving of attempted and failed abortions, knows that its presence is resented and its life in danger.

It relives its own near murder, terror of death, with quite astounding accuracy. The enormous feelings of rejection throughout adult life are an affliction for many who have survived this horror. The near miss of a spontaneous abortion can leave the threat of doom around the corner as a permanent memory. Also the preborn can pick up mother's terror and make it their own, so there is a double terror.

Accidents

Accidents to the pregnant mother, like falling down stairs, car and bicycle crashes, may also appear to the foetus as attempts to kill. Baby logic, when arising in the adult, may be quite misplaced and regression work can rectify the picture which has become misplaced by the adult.

The Death Of A Twin

The loss of a twin in utero is more common than can be imagined, and mother may or may not be aware of this, but the remaining foetus does know. Only about 40% of zygotes will find a secure place in the lining of the womb. Some are spontaneously aborted before finding a secure place, so in this way conceptions fail before the mother even knows she is pregnant. This can be very stressful to clients reliving the loss of a twin or even triplets. The guilt on the surviving twin is enormous and the blame is heavy. The desire may be to return where the twin has gone, as the pain of separation is too great.

The Loss Of An Identical Twin

One client not only recalled the loss of an identical twin in the womb, but also a third embryo, which is a multiple conception. Althea Hayton in her book *Womb Twin Survivors* explains that the sole survivors of a multiple conception tend to re-enact their own womb story in intimate relationships by co-dependency and self-absorption. She explains how the multiple womb twin survivor has a tendency to sabotage relationships, which re-enacts the original pre-birth tragedy.

There is a correlation here with intra-uterine events causing schizoid personality disorder as in identical twin survivors where there is a feeling of being split in two, yet there is only one individual left alive. Hayton describes this as self-absorption and states that in the *Dream of the Womb* there is someone very close by and exactly the same. This part of the self is very vulnerable and fragile and needs constant and absolute attention, so all energy is directed inwardly.

The Schizoid Personality - Case Study

The dominant script of the client reliving this scenario was one of feeling very fragile, small and possessing a great fear of annihilation. The adult had a great need to protect their own traumatised child—*the vanished twin*—keeping the child alive by adopting the schizoid, closed, defensive position, and in one sense, completely ignoring the lost twin. In her inner life this client believed that if she stopped trying to keep herself alive she would dissolve into nothingness and vanish—just like her identical *vanished* twin.

The Umbilical Effect

Frank Lake's theories are vindicated, but this work suggests that awareness goes back even further, even to implantation and before. It is at the joining up of the now functioning foetal circulation with that of the mother, with a finger placed on the navel in a regression session, to stimulate the cord, that the *umbilical affect* is powerfully experienced, whether negative or positive.

Signs Of The Journey From Fallopian Tube To Uterus

As the next stage in our journey back to conception, this chapter will take us from the attempts to implant on the wall of the womb, back to the journey made down the fallopian tube by the fertilized egg in its earliest stage as a blastocyst.

Implantation

The scripts that come from implantation have surprised us over the years. We have been going further and further back in utero in order to find the healing places for people. Although this is not necessary for everyone, it does help to know that if reliving the birth trauma does not heal the problem then it is possible to keep going further back. This is not uncommon with those familiar with Grof's work.

Implantation is the first time we connect physically with mother. As in the fusion of the sperm and ovum, the fertilised ovum may find a resistant uterine wall. Implantation actually does involve fingerlike projections of foetal tissue that take root in the wall of the uterus. Finding a place to implant in the womb has an effect on the way in which people fit into life.

Scripts from implantation are:

I have no place to be.
I can't settle anywhere.
I'm in the wrong place. I don't belong anywhere.
Nobody wants me here. I am half-afraid to aim for anything.
Why does it have to be so hard to find a comfortable place.
Out of one bloody mess into another one.

To find one's place in life is vital and to find a place of belonging is part of the healing process of therapy. It is an interesting factor to relive how one found one's safety and security in the womb.

Difficulty in implantation, and a desperation to find a place to be, can culminate in adult life as never finding the right place to be, and the isolation may drive the person to suicide, for in adult life the terrible isolation can be overwhelming.

The Mother's Attitude To The Pregnancy

When mother finds out she is pregnant and the response is negative, the whole organism feels:

I shouldn't be here
It's all my fault
I'll end it as I'm the cause of her distress

We have taken our clients back in regression to preconception and conception, and discovered information relating to the emotional state of the parents-to-be and the situation awaiting the incoming soul.

Frank Lake emphasised four levels of responses by the baby in utero and also around birth:-

Ideally Good where all is well in the respective parents to be, there is no stress, there is passionate lovemaking and a real focus of wanting a baby. It is interesting to note that rarely, if at all, people who may have experienced this blissful situation before conception, actually appear in therapy.

Bearing and Coping and *mild anger* may be present if a *tired* sperm and *fairly reluctant* ovum find it difficult to fertilise in a *lethargic* or *can't be bothered* environment—but it is *good enough* and self-confidence is present.

Total Opposition—where there is no desire to conceive a child. Here the anger and terror may be paramount in the mother or father. It is a bad place. No preparation for conception, which will in turn attract rejection and hostility toward the new individual.

Transmarginal Stress—Before conception there are overwhelming feelings of badness and bitterness relating to possible lust, anger, rape and drunkenness. Here is beyond the margin, stress beyond bearing—everything to do with fighting has become too painful to bear. Here is the root of the most determined refusal to seek life or let oneself be loved. It is from the experiences of levels three and four that many angry situations arise.

Parental Consciousness

Bonding begins before conception, in the relationship between mother and father and at the moment of conception that bonding may be sealed. The consciousness of each of the parents, and their feelings at that moment of conception continues to be in the energy in and around the womb throughout pregnancy. Furthermore, the attachment patterns we form in early life stay with us and are generally re-enacted in all later relationships, most especially intimate ones. Any traumatic experience between pre—conception and birth where bonding is threatened, cut off or has never been sealed, will cause dysfunction at the level of the trauma experienced.

In our most recent research we believe that very early parent—ing begins before conception. If our discoveries and experiences in Pre and Perinatal Psychotherapy are to be taken seriously, then the state of the parents to be is of immense importance to the well being of the new individual to be conceived.

If we are affected in infancy, childhood and adulthood by the positive and negative situations in our life—then it appears from regression work that the sexual act between our parents, in what—ever emotions or non-emotions we were conceived, will affect our coming into being.

Pre-Conception Life Scripts

We have, through visualisation, artwork, regression and primal work been able to help hundreds of clients *tune in* to the emotional state of their mothers and fathers before conception. Many of the feelings experienced through visualisation etc., come through the feelings of being the ovum or the sperm, and what happens as they meet and fertilise. The anger, violence and outrage that unwanted conceptions relive in regression together with the fear of rejection is also a very frequent part of their personality in adult life and is projected on many people and *rejection felt* situations in life. It is such a painful place to live from, it may turn inwards into great internal anger that eventually violates the body and causes sickness. Some scripts are:-

It was a violent scene. They physically enjoyed it but the sperm is an onslaught. The ovum was emotionally raped.

I'm really angry. My conception was an accident and I've had accidents ever since. I battle with my mother continually.

It's all very difficult. The sperm is full of life, it's energetic and playful. It wants to connect. It wants to penetrate the ovum. It wants to connect. The ovum is so rigid. It's so resistant.

It's a huge struggle for the sperm to get in. But it got in at last.

Birth trauma is an event that reverberates throughout life, acting like a fractal that constantly replicates itself, but this chapter has shown that the time before birth can also be a source of trauma.

The pre-birth memory is remarkably precise and is related to the particular time in the womb when the trauma occurred. The mysteries of prenatal consciousness are becoming clearer as we regress more and more clients to the earliest time of their existence. The next chapter will provide some longer case studies, which will answer some questions but present still more mysteries to be understood—but then that has always been the nature of our work at Amethyst.

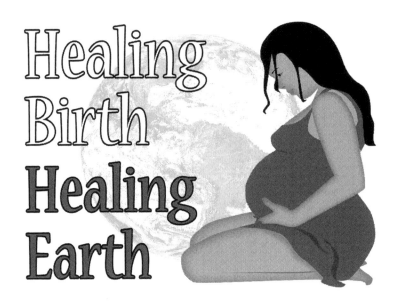

PART THREE

Chapter 9

SOME CASE STUDIES

PRE- AND PERINATAL WORK WITH INFANTS AND CHILDREN

Medical Intervention During Pregnancy

Carmel Byrne is the Child and Adolescent Psychotherapist at Amethyst and has supplied the following case studies:

Wendy: Pete and Margaret's three year old daughter Wendy was a blonde, beautiful, blue-eyed girl, an only child. They knew of the work I do with children on healing birth, using play therapy, toys, sand tray work, art, puppets, games and other creative methods. Although Wendy was only three, they brought her because they were worried about her withdrawn behaviour.

Mother brought Wendy for a session, having already sent me correspondence concerning Wendy's behavioural problems. Wendy would not allow anyone to touch her, not even her father or mother. Wendy was fine if no-one touched her. If anyone tried to touch or hold her she would go into sheer panic, turn white and run away and hide.

I asked mother about Wendy's birth and she responded that Wendy was born on her due date, it was only four hours labour and was a natural birth with no drugs.

I was a little apprehensive as to where to start with Wendy as she stood across the room and just looked at me. I decided to include mother in the session in s different way. As she stood in the corner of the room, Wendy would not leave her corner. Mother tried to coax her out but all was in vain. I decided to make a swimming pool with the large cushions in the room and invite Wendy's mum to come and join me to have some fun. We pretended to enjoy the swimming pool and made quite a lot of noise between us as we were playing.

Suddenly Wendy started to scream and went blue in the face. Mother was frightened and went over immediately to comfort her, which made the situation worse. I went over but stayed a distance away from Wendy to give her space. I spoke to her assuring her that I knew it hurt a lot and I was sorry that it was so painful for her. I told her I would like to help her and be her friend. I also promised I wouldn't come any nearer but she could tell me how near I could go to her.

Wendy had stopped crying and was looking at me. Mother was very upset and Wendy said, *"Mammy's sad."*

I kept my full attention on Wendy as she stood there looking very lost, afraid and lonely. She made eye contact with me for a while and I could see her eyes were full of fear, as if she were on guard in case anyone came near to her.

In the next session Wendy ventured a little nearer to me. She had something to show me. Mother had taken her to the toy shop and Wendy would not leave until she had bought a doctor's set, which contained all sorts of medical instruments.

I asked Wendy if she would like to play a game of doctors and nurses. To my surprise she agreed. She said she wanted to be the doctor and I was to be sick. So I lay down and Wendy started to take my temperature and told me to stay in bed as I was sick.

Suddenly Wendy started to scream again, shouting and trembling with fear. She threw away the doctor's set and when I came towards her she had a forceps type of instrument in her hand, and still screaming she threw it at me. Her words amidst the screams were,

"They are hurting me!"
"Get them away from me!"
"Help! Help! Help!"
"Mammy! Mammy! Mammy!"
"Wendy don't like that!"
"Wendy afraid!"
"Help Wendy!"
"It's hurting me"
"I want to get away from it."

She pushed herself up against the wall as if she were trying to escape through it. She pointed to the back of her neck and head complaining of being very sore. I asked if I could help to make it better for her and maybe she would come over to me. She did and turned her back on her mammy and me, to show her head and neck. There were marks on her neck as if some sharp pointed instrument had been stuck into her. With her mammy standing close by, I stroked Wendy's neck gently and she went into a full cathartic experience. She then walked quietly away and sat and played on the cushions.

We had five sessions of play therapy and five sessions for integration.

Mother eventually told me that she was five months pregnant before she discovered she was carrying Wendy. Her periods were irregular and she believed she had a medical problem. She went to the doctors who gave her a full examination using a medical instrument. Mother's intuition was that this was the event that had probably traumatised her baby in the womb and was responsible for Wendy's problematic behaviour.

Both Pete and Margaret were amazed and astounded that Wendy insisted on being given the doctors set at the toy shop and even more amazed at her reaction to the instrument she was so upset about, which took her into reliving the intrusion into her space in the womb.

As the ten sessions drew to a close, Wendy relaxed and allowed closeness to me and her mammy and daddy. They were delighted with her progress and she was by then a happy little girl attending a Montessori School.

Foetal Alcohol Syndrome (FAS)

Andy: Andy was nearly 6 years old when his GP referred him to me. He had already seen a psychologist, a psychiatrist and a speech and language therapist. His mother was Irish, a single mother with her own addiction to alcohol and drugs. She was also in court for petty crimes and had her own psychological problems. Father was from the Far East with his own addiction problems and had little or no contact with Andy. Andy's school gave him a lot of help trying to keep him and the other children safe from Andy's serious behaviour problems. The teachers tried to contain him but reported nothing worked and he was passed from one professional to another. When his sessions began I found him to be very nervous and scattered in his behaviour but he was polite, intelligent and with a very strong will. He shared a great deal with me and said he punched and kicked the other children because they called him names. Although he was born in Ireland he looked different from them.

He worked using art, the sand tray and storytelling. In art he would always draw monsters coming to get him, but before they did he would get them first. He worked his anger out in sound. He had to punch and kick the monster before it hurt him. He was terrified of being hit and punched and kicked and this behaviour came out in him when others were angry with him. He was frightened of aggression, and verbal and physical abuse. As the sessions continued there appeared to be signs of FAS–Foetal Alcohol Syndrome. Mother confirmed that she was drinking alcohol during her pregnancy. FAS is now scientifically and medically proven. Andy showed the following symptoms relating to FAS:

non-compliant behaviour
unable to follow instructions
very anxious
easily frustrated by the actions of other children
not able to wait in line or for his turn
required constant supervision
destructive behaviour
stands close to people like 'in your face'
lengthy temper tantrums
oppositional—if you say, 'Yes' then he will say, 'No'

The extremes in his behaviour were very difficult to deal with; not able to sit still, fidgets, wiggles and squirms and is very easily over-stimulated. Andy was also unable to make connections between actions and consequences.

The Work Begins

In his sessions, Andy decided he wanted to lie down under a table with cushions all around him. This went on for 15 sessions when he was able to display his anger, fear and frustration and he stayed in this position for up to 40 minutes.

He commented that in this place he was in sticky water and the sticky water was coming to get him. It had a bad smell, he could taste it in his mouth. He would go into a panic shouting for help and saying he was going to die, that he hated her and she was going to kill him. If she did not stop and let him out he would kill her. After these experiences he would come out and say, *"I feel better."*

After 16 sessions the school reported that Andy was improving greatly, his behaviour was manageable and he was listening more.

I slowly introduced another child into the sessions which at first was unacceptable to Andy, but little by little he started to share the toys. The school then came on board and cooperated by involving Andy into group projects in plays and school outings. They introduced him to art, music and sport in which he excelled. He was able to interact with others and learned to control his anger and direct it to be creative and not destructive.

He left primary school and made an easier transition than the teachers thought he would, to go to the secondary school. He obtained 10 A-levels in the Junior Cert and is now studying for his Leaving Certificate. By re-experiencing his time in the womb where he was marinated in alcohol he had the courage and determination to face his problems and have a better quality of life.

He is now able to meet the challenges of life without the baggage of his early life. His mother's problems are improving and Andy spends a lot of time with his dad.

Umbilical Cord & Family Crises

Bobby: Bobby was 7 years old when his parents brought him to me for help. His sister Rebecca was just 14 months older than him. His parents wanted a brother or sister for him because they lived out in the country and there were no children living nearby to play with. Mother explained that Bobby was very clingy and would not leave her side; he was very scared of loud voices and would jump at the slightest sound and movement. He was unable to bond to anyone and was terrified of being hurt. He found it hard to sleep at night and had night terrors. When he cried, he would do so for up to six hours without stopping.

Mother had taken him to a number of professionals but I was her last hope, as her intuition was telling her that Bobby's problems were due to the family crises during and around her pregnancy with him. When mum and dad found they were pregnant with Bobby they were overjoyed. The pregnancy was fine; mum had a little morning sickness but nothing else. However, the external crises surrounding them when they were pregnant with Bobby were devastatingly stressful. There was no money to pay bills, dad lost his job, they were on the point of losing the house and moved in with her mother. Dad was grieving owing to the loss of both his parents in a short time and his sense of failure and shame drove him to attempt to take his own life by overdosing on tablets, but he was found in time and survived.

The night of Bobby's birth mum felt unwell after eating a large meal so she went to bed. She felt a lot of pressure about 11pm and asked her husband to get the ambulance. At this point her mother came home from the pub drunk. She was screaming and shouting in a drunken frenzy telling them to stop the ambulance from coming. On arrival at the hospital the midwives would not allow her husband in. Mother was still screaming and shouting in the corridor in her drunken stupor so much that security removed her from the hospital.

Bobby's mum was very upset as she had wanted a calm and peaceful birth for her baby. Instead there was chaos, screaming and shouting and crisis after crisis; nurses ignoring her and no husband allowed in to comfort her. In the end Bobby was pulled out by forceps, his face was damaged and cut, and the cord was round his neck. The nurses took him away for four days and put him into an incubator. Neither mother or father saw their son for four days.

He was brought back four days later, for his mother to breast feed him, which she couldn't do and in the end she rejected her own son.

When I first met Bobby I was expecting him to be withdrawn like so many children but he came into the room, and at 7 years of age shook my hand and said he was pleased to meet me. His mother had told him he was going to meet a lady who was going to help him. With Bobby's initial reaction I felt he was ready for his journey into his birth. He started to play with the cushions, made a tunnel and asked his mother to cover him up with them.

Immediately mother's instincts that his problems were due to the environment of his birth began to be proved right. At first under the cushions he said he was fine but continued to say that he didn't like this place as it was cold, dark and noisy. He was very scared and said that he couldn't do it as he was not going to get it right, he hated the dark and liked to sleep with the light on.

Asked if he would like his mother to take the cushions off he firmly said, *"No"*. As they would all see him. Using the Gestalt method, I suggested to Bobby that he asked the tunnel questions. He asked the tunnel what was going to be done to him and was he going to die. He wanted to know why he was being trapped inside, what all the noise was about and what was going to happen next. He pleaded with the tunnel not to hurt him or choke him as he could feel something round his neck. Asking for help he said he would be very good as he was so scared he needed someone to love him.

Bobby eventually popped out, looked around and asked if he was really in the room all the time. He thought he was really trapped somewhere, couldn't get out and was going to die.

When he returned for another session he came in with his mam saying that he needed to go back into the tunnel and cushions. Going in, he immediately told his mother to please, please stop the noise and the fighting. This continued for a number of sessions where he was able to find the words to express himself. After this process Bobby became more compliant, went to friend's house for overnight stays which he would never do before. His fears of getting close to people became less. Noise was now not a problem and he was able to ask for help. He began to trust his parents who were delighted with the change in him. On finishing his sessions Bobby said to me,

"Carmel, I am glad I came to see you. I now feel free. I can fly and I am not afraid."

Chapter 10

PRE- AND PERINATAL WORK WITH ADULTS

Pre- And Perinatal Work With Adults

Frank Lake's hypothesis that all patterns are there from conception and colour our life and the rhythms and patterns of our lives are formed from that early fusion, are being experienced in the therapy room. The energy fusion at conception in our life cycle from cell one, seems to absorb and store that original energy pattern.

Whatever is happening between the mother and her baby in the nine-month pre-birth period, the interactions between them will extend into childhood and beyond. The projections of negative womb experiences become irrational behaviour whilst positive experiences develop into a better adapted human being. For healing to take place these prebirth primal experiences acquire the emotional, physical sensation and historical memory.

The following case studies from courageous people show how their prebirth scripts brought into consciousness the origins of their problems and help them transform their lives.

Patsy

I was a home birth in Ireland in the 1950's. I arrived head first and according to mother I came head first, did it all myself and *did it right*. So I was a *normal* birth, whatever that means, but devastating things happened to me before I took my first breath of oxygen. In therapy I would sit in the chair saying nothing, but being completely unaware that my distress was preverbal. I was at a loss for words, the feelings were in my body but I was unable to access them. I felt trapped with no way out and wanted to be discovered.

Since experiencing pre- and perinatal work I have discovered a backdrop against which to view my experiences and with that comes a lot of understanding and insights. This was helped by therapy I had done on myself previously. I always felt there were secrets in my life. My secrets are about letting people know who I am. Yet the desire to be discovered goes side by side with the fear of annihilation if I am found out. I had so much physical pain, a pain to be someone—lately to be me is sufficient.

My secrets go back a long way. My mother did not want to believe that she was pregnant and I did not want to believe that I existed.

She had a secret and I became a secret. In adult life I have found reality hard to take and use all manner of avoidance, and if it doesn't work I spontaneously go blank and it has been a difficult and painful struggle to keep in touch with reality. I left the country for two years, trying to run away and avoid the pain but it went with me and I returned disillusioned and in despair. My mother concealed her pregnancy. I have a tendency to hide, to hide my feelings, my knowledge and my existence. My mother felt shame as her body began to grow with me. I feel shame when I put on weight.

In therapy I experienced my time in utero as being in a toxic womb. My mother had been advised not to have any more children as she suffered from high blood pressure. She was frightened during the pregnancy especially towards the end. My mother's fear became my fear. My life in the womb was a life lived in constant fear. To escape this unbearable time I dissociated from the pain but it also became my companion. Because there was nothing of a nourishing nature coming through the cord I learned to exist in pain. Later in life I know that my self-injurious behaviour came directly from this place. In utero, backing away from the cord has given me a spinal weakness. I was born with the cord around my neck, lost consciousness and nearly died.

From experiencing pre- and perinatal psychotherapy and becoming aware of these primal origins I have begun to know my real self. I did not know that I had the right to choose in life. I did not have a voice. The re-experiencing the first nine months of my life has given me to myself. I have come a long way on my journey. May my journey ahead continue on the sacred path of healing and transformation.

Annie

Although I love life now, for my earlier years of life I was unfortunate enough to be conceived out of wedlock in Catholic Ireland in the 1950's. The fear and anxiety that she went through were so excruciating that during my therapy sessions I felt myself dissociate and split off. My mother was firstly given the choice to go into a mother and baby home or vanish to England. But her mother then insisted she go to England rather than bring more shame on the family. I was growing and being marinated in all these negative emotions.

Although she stayed in England and kept me the feelings in me of shame and profound fear and lack of trust in men have caused huge problems in my life.

I have enormous difficulty maintaining close friends and relationships and an impending sense that if people find out what a terrible person I am they will not want to know me. My father eventually joined her but their sense of having done such a terrible thing with my forthcoming birth affected me in a way that I became the *foetal therapist*. I tried to detach from my own experiences and then look after everyone else.

The therapeutic work that I have done is helping me make great changes in my life and I am now in a loving relationship. When the time comes I will know when I need to do further work. In some ways I wish I had found the therapy years earlier but now knowing the origins of my problems explored in pre- and perinatal work has given me hope for the future.

Peter

In my life I have carried many patterns or scripts and one of the major ones being, *anything is better than staying where I am.* I recognise I still operate from this premise. I had little information about my birth but relations told me my mother was very frightened and was in labour for over 16 hours. My mother had contracted Multiple Sclerosis prior to my conception and was told by doctors not to have children as she might die giving birth or be left paralysed. I was her first, and only, baby and the reason for the long labour was due to the fact that she was too frightened to let me go and literally held me back for over 12 hours. This led to a life script for me of,

I am paralysed and stuck and don't know what is going to happen next.

This is a present day life script. In therapy I have experienced strong feelings of paralysis and fear in conception, in the womb and birth as well. Running deep through my life there has been a script of,

I must hang on or I will be swept away.

In my adult life, giving birth to change and implementing it, are long drawn out affairs, filled with fear and apprehension of *what might happen*. The model or energy was laid down at birth and before. Prior to therapy I would have lived in a *paralysed process* hoping change would happen rather than making it happen. The legacy of my birth experience has been my crucifixion and resurrection.

I have through many years of self-exploration at last found the keys of understanding how I am and who I am. I can seek in a positive fashion to find new ways of moving from this place of acknowledgement and recognition.

My birth and life fit into the global scale of what has been happening to our history experience of the 20th Century. This has been a century of birth, a time of recognising the pain of past patterns, as in Europe, with war, and a time of reconstruction and moving forward from the old scripts of isolation and domination to co-operation and expansion of this century's story. You and I who live now are part of this shifting, changing story where the shifts and changes in our individual lives feed into the energy of total consciousness.

Fallopian Tube Trauma

Susan:

It was seven or eight years since I had seen my therapist and after I had experienced my life in the womb I went home and got on with living! I had mastered the changes and knowledge necessary to improve my quality of life.

Something else was preventing me to move further on a deeper level. I was getting stuck in life, particularly in relationships and developing projects that as a creative artist I wished to pursue in the future. I was also suffering from low blood pressure which was debilitating when I tried to put more energy into shifting projects forward. I told my therapist it felt completely irrational but it certainly felt it came from an earlier period of birth and the forceps delivery I encountered at birth. This is what happened when I lay down on the mattress in her room and closed my eyes:

Therapist: Where are you?
Susan: I feel very small. I feel like a tiny ball in a tube. My head is swirling. I feel sick. I'm somewhere but I'm nowhere. The pain is in my chest. It's just like the feelings I have when my blood pressure drops.

Th: But it's not your blood pressure here.
S: OK. But it is the same feeling I get when my blood pressure drops.

Th: When you feel your head swirl how long does it last?
S: It feels forever.

Th: Where does it feel?
S: In my chest but it also feels right through me.

Th: What shape are you?
S: I feel like the shape of a marble but it is not hard like a marble. I feel round.

Th: So, you are round. Where do you feel the swirling in you?
S: Right through me. It's black. And the feeling makes me sick.

Th: How long does this sickness last when you get it?
S: It feels forever but I'm stuck. I feel fragile like a dandelion seed.

Th: You're fragile. Like a dandelion?

S: Yes but I'm stuck. I don't know what to do. I'm round—but I don't feel the right shape to go through, or to go where I am supposed to go.

Th: Which way are you going?

S: That way. (Pointing to feet) I'm not the right shape I'll never get where I'm going. I can't decide. I shouldn't be thinking here. It's not right to think here. This should be happening naturally and spontaneously.

Th: So it's not your fault that you're stuck?

S: No. But nobody is helping. I shouldn't be stuck here. Something there should be moving. (Hands wave in front) Something should be helping me along but something outside is paralysed. She's paralysed. Her tension is stopping me. It's not me. It's not my fault. But if I stay here I shall die.

Th: It's something from outside that's stopping you. When you feel this stopping you, how long does it stop you for?

S: Forever. It feels like I'll never get through. I can't decide what to do. I don't know which way to go. I'm just round, like a round small ball. I should know which way to go—this is ridiculous. The tension inside is dreadful.

Th: When you get this tension how long does it last?

S: It's always there. It's like I shall explode. It's not physical. It's a mental tension.

Th: So it's a mental tension? What will happen if you explode?

S: I shall die. I've got so much energy to get moving but something outside is stopping me and it isn't me. It's out there. (Rocking movements)

Th: What will happen if you move?

S: It's dreadful. The swirling. I have got to get through to where I am going. But I am frightened of what is going to happen. I'm stuck. It feels like any minute I could die. I am not going to make it, I can't move forward in the dark and I can't go back to the light.

Th: Where would you go to if you went back into the light?

S: It's good but I can't go back. I'm stuck. I'm here. There should be movement. Something's happening. I feel like I am turning like a ball. But it is not a round ball like a marble that goes straight it's like one of those beach balls with panels, you roll it but it doesn't go straight. I feel dizzy and sick. I've moved a bit but I'm frightened. I feel like I am going to shoot forward. Very fast.

Th: If you shoot forward very fast what will happen?

S: I won't be able to cope.

Th: Has something changed?

S: Yes! I'm moving. See I'm doing it. I'm too big. I've stayed too long. I can't get through (real fear and panic) I'm too big. I need help. The pressure inside is awful. I feel sick. She's not relaxing, God there is so much tension out there. I have got to do this. (Real push to move forward.) I'm doing it I'm going to make it. That's better. I am still in the tube but I'm freer. More space. It's a bigger area. There's something ahead of me that I'm afraid of—but I'm freer.

Th: The important thing is you did it. You didn't need help. I didn't have to help you. You did it.

S: Yes that feels good. I did it. I can do it!

The journey of my birth through the birth canal was a fractal of my journey through the fallopian tube. I obviously needed to go back further to dissipate early trauma that was so deeply instilled that it caused me distress. I was aware that my mother conceived during the Second World War during the bombing of London where they lived. The external environment of war has devastating effects upon the unborn.

After experiencing this very early journey in the fallopian tube my low blood pressure improved and I had the incentive and energy to move forward in life. I began to love the speed of aeroplanes, motor bikes and fast cars and travelled to different countries whenever I could.

An amusing thing is, as a child I hated funfairs and spinning rides, they made me sick, and no way could my parents get me to the funfair for a treat! Also in the early days of driving a car, when having parked a car in the car park I could never find the way out of the car park! Now I love fast cars and can never get to Disneyland or funfairs fast enough!

Giving Birth To Change - My Story

In my adult life giving birth to change and implementing it, are long drawn out affairs, filled with fear and apprehension of *what might happen*. The model or energy was laid down at birth and before. Prior to therapy I would have lived in a *paralysed process* hoping change would happen rather than making it happen. The legacy of my birth experience has been my crucifixion and resurrection. I have, through many years of self-exploration at last found the keys of understanding how I am, who I am, and I can seek in a positive fashion to find new ways of moving from this place of acknowledgement and recognition. On a global scale, this is what has been happening to our history experience of the 20th century. It has been a century of birth, a time of recognising the pain of past patterns (i.e. in Europe—war), a time of reconstruction and a time of moving forward from the old scripts of isolation and domination to co-operation and expansion of this century's story.

You and I who live now are part of this shifting, changing story where the change and shifts in our individual lives feed into the energy of total consciousness. Each individual's story and experience is part of the 'great story' of the human experience. In many ways although each of our individual lives differ we all contribute to the great consciousness of human experience. We are a global family and 'space ship earth' is our home. We have ultimately been born from the stars and now in this age we strive to return to our origins.There is a parallel connection between our journey to the stars (seeking our origins?) and now seeking to journey back to birth, conception and beyond. It is as if the human consciousness is seeking a new way to live and *be* in the desire to revisit our origins.

In this new millennium there is a yearning in an age of healing for the individual, healing for the nations and healing for the planet. A yearning for wholeness and a new way to be. My dream is that I will contribute and be part of the time to come and that I will make a difference.

Chapter 11

EXPERIENTIAL THERAPY

Carrie - Case Study

This case study illustrating work we carried out at Amethyst in 1993, is one that clearly shows how Frank Lake's hypotheses of ten to twenty years ago were valid. This work was videoed in one of our primal integration and regression therapy training groups. It also relates to our hypothesis that the human body remembers everything that has ever happened to it and that these memories can and will surface.

Carrie had done a lot of regression work previously, so this was not her first experience. She was a recovering sufferer from ME (Myalgic Encephalomyeltis), known in the US as Chronic Fatigue Syndrome.

Carrie found she was splitting her energies by living and working in two places—Belfast in Northern Ireland and Dublin in the South—because she was not sure where she wanted to be. She was also wanting to make a commitment to a relationship and was finding it difficult.

Before her practical work Carrie talked about living in Belfast. She expressed a certain heaviness about there and a freedom in being able to come to Dublin as well. She was also afraid she was going to get stuck!

"I enjoy living there but I've always had a sense of not wanting to be there. I'm fine here at the moment but in the future I'm going to be somewhere else!"

I asked Carrie what she felt she would like to change in her life.

"I have been in shock for a long time. I feel frozen. I want to be free."

Preconception

As the session began, Carrie experienced preconception.

"My body feels like it doesn't belong to me. I just feel like I am swirling. I am just all energy. It's like being in a dark vortex."

When asked if there was any purpose in this dark vortex,

"I'm being drawn into something."

Conception

Asked by Alison: *"Can you discover what you are being drawn into?"*

Carrie: *"Something is happening now. I'm being drawn into somewhere I don't want to go. It's dark—it's like I'm somewhere but I'm nowhere."*

There were many flickering, shuddering movements of her body, similar to those that Dr. William Emerson and Dr. Graham Farrant have spoken of in the past and believe to be very early movements.

"I think I'm waiting for something to happen and I don't know what ..."

The body shuddering and foot movements continued for some time. When asked, *"Have you a shape or form yet—or are you still a vortex of energy?"* her response was, *"I'm round"*.

Experience As The Fertilised Ovum

"I'm trying to fit into something that is too small. It's like a shell."

She was asked, *"What is it like being confined inside this shell that is too small for you?"* She replied, *"It's safe and too confined and I want to break out."*

In The Fallopian Tube

"I'm in a passage—sometimes I move—sometimes I don't."

Awareness Of Twin Sister

"There is something behind me. It feels like somebody else. They are getting further away. I don't want to leave her behind."

Womb Awareness

"Where are you now?"

"I'm in a big space like a cave."

Implantation

When asked if it was a nice space, Carrie responded that she was getting comfortable and her physical body moved into a comfortable position representing implantation.

Waiting For Sister's Arrival

"I can't concentrate! I'm waiting for her to arrive. It's not comfortable any more. There's a beautiful blue light. She's over there—she's my sister."

Awareness Of Cord

"I have a cord—it's too big!" When asked what was coming through the cord she replied, *"She's afraid* (mother*). I think she is afraid she's pregnant. I'm four weeks now. It's all coming in."*

Spontaneous Abortion Of Another Embryo

"I'm seven weeks. There's something wrong." With distress and grief, *"She's going, she won't stay, she's giving up. I think she's fading out."*

The therapist empathising, says: *"And you hurt, don't you?"*

Mother's Emotions

"She's sad. She's peaceful."

Alison says, *"There's an awful lot that's happened to you so far in the first eight weeks of life."*

Carrie Discussing Her Work The Next Day

Carrie's session lasted one and a half hours. She explained:

"I think I'm still shell-shocked. The most significant period was the first 8 weeks, and the feeling of being energy. I was very aware of two energies. It shocked me. For the moment it (conception energy) was like an invasion—it was so sudden. It was like I had to squeeze all my energy into something small. I want freedom. I want space. I am not wanting to be constricted. I want to move."

From her work, Carrie will need to integrate the shock that came in at conception and the fragmented energies. The loss of a twin as far back as in the fallopian tube or the first few weeks in the womb could be the roots of commitment anxiety combined with the fear of separation. There is much food for thought in Carrie's work and many points for discussion.

Chapter 12

EXPERIENTIAL PSYCHOTHERAPY
HEALING SUICIDAL FEELINGS

Memories & Feelings

Looking for that which is not visible is at the foundation of pre- and perinatal psychotherapy when working with those who are suffering the excruciating pain that can be at the primal roots of suicidal tendencies.

At Amethyst we work with clients in a variety of ways: perinatal psychotherapy, primal integration, regression therapy, energy healing, visualisation, meditation, art work, shamanic journeying, music, gestalt and other humanistic and integrative therapies.

Pre- and perinatal psychology is dedicated to the in-depth exploration of the psychological dimension of human reproduction and pregnancy. Within all these complicated issues of humanity are those of suicide and attempted suicide. It is my belief that at any point during the conception, pregnancy or birth, where the pain of the single cell, the blastocyst, the foetus, the preborn, is beyond the point of bearing, suicidal thoughts and tendencies take their roots.

The Retrieval Of Pre- and Perinatal Memories

The retrieval of pre- and perinatal memories, from before and around birth, and including as far back as conception, can help us understand how and why we behave as we do in the world. The deep parenting and spiritual parenting of our own self discovery of those primal times, begins to heal what might have gone amiss in the conception, gestation and birth from our physical parents.

Remembering helps the re-creation of us. It creates the deep healing of what went wrong—and the deepening realisation of what went right.

It is important to remember and experience the positive, in order to empower our whole being and to overcome negative blocks, which have hampered the development of human potential. Many answers are found in these periods of human development, the study of which are still in the infancy stage.

Studying Birth And Intra-Uterine Memories

Today researchers are studying birth and intra-uterine memories and movements from two perspectives. Firstly, scientific studies of the activities of the unborn and newborn baby are being documented, particularly the unborn, with the use of ultra sound scanning of the foetus in utero. So from before birth ultrasound is revealing the hidden life of the unborn baby.

The second perspective is that of birth and womb experiences relived by adults, children and babies in regression therapies or other body related therapies and hypnosis. It is through the experiential work that the following stories are told.

Healing Suicidal Feelings

Ann (1980)

Ann writes: On reflection I had a severe schizoid personality disorder. It caused me such great distress and pain that it was easier for me to cut off from the pain than allow myself to feel the suffering at a deep level. Consequently I lived my life at a superficial level and the pain was well hidden. But at times when it surfaced and became intolerable I wanted to die. I first attempted suicide at the age of thirteen with an overdose of pills. At the time I had no idea why I had done this—but parental illness, my own physical pain and family financial pressures caused intolerable responsibilities that I was too young to deal with. I had thought about ending it all, many times.

My own regression work as an adult took me to the earliest places in my life when I experienced the primal pain of rejection through attempted abortion, more than once, and the most horrific forceps delivery that felt like it was severing my head from my body. I had no idea that my therapy would take me into these places and I certainly had no knowledge that the human organism was capable of remembering so far back.

But the feelings that used to rack through my body every time I went into new situations took me into reliving my birth situation of rejection, fear and horror of not being wanted. I could relate superficially but wanted no closeness. I always sat close to doors and windows in a room—I realised later it was a way of escape if people got too close. I often wanted help from others but spurned it. I felt I needed help but no way would accept it and became known as a very independent individual.

But underneath the pain were intolerable feelings of rejection and annihilation—caused by the attempted abortions—which eventually led to very fast car driving, and car accidents, which thankfully involved no-one else, and did not kill me or anyone else, although unconsciously I now know the suicide attempts were there.

I am aware that therapists may be filled with empathy and compassion but be baffled why a certain individual experiences herself at the core of her being as so utterly wretched and worthless.

But finding out either from mother or the client experiencing what mother's feelings were, when she realised in shocked recognition that she was pregnant has had a terrible impact on the growing foetus. That this new life was a disaster which mother both feared and hated intensely, and mother's feelings transfusing the foetus, who often is aware of being a loathed object and not a person, are other places during pregnancy which have a devastating personality affect, all of which becomes projected onto present day life.

My own feelings of suicide were illogical but after reliving the trauma and stress of the pregnancy and birth I realised there was a real place in life from where these feelings came. This was the healing. The change of behaviour came from knowing I was not mad. It was no-one's fault. There was no-one to blame. At that time my parents did not know that anything negative that was happening in their lives was coming into me.

I no longer have suicidal feelings because they do not belong in the present. I was meant to live—not die young. But if I had not learned the primal place where these feelings had originally come from I would have died by suicide over twenty-five years ago. I understand that with this prenatal distress percolating into adult life it is no wonder these early primal events are projected and cause suicidal tendencies.

Healing Suicidal Feelings: Sarah (2003)

A more recent experience of discovering where suicidal feelings originate. This young woman has only recently discovered the origin of her feelings of suicide and wanting to die.

In telling you my story, and my struggle to both live and die, it involves the struggle to survive my inheritance from both my parents. My fight has been to break the cycle, not only for my sake, but also for the sake of my children.

My mother had a history of difficult births, and I was the seventh. My mother's first delivery almost ended in her death. Her life hung in the balance for almost a week following an emergency caesarian. I was 10lbs 11ozs in weight and was delivered by forceps. In retrospect I lived my childhood in the shadow of fear.

As I entered puberty, life was going to get worse. Life began to terrify me. It was terrible. My fear intensified and I was afraid to move in case I moved the wrong way. At the age of 16, a year after taking my first drink I began to suffer from depression.

I couldn't figure out what was happening to me and I decided that life was not worth living and I had my first suicide attempt—overdosing on aspirin. I was in such emotional pain and didn't know how to deal with it. My only way of killing this pain was either to get drunk or overdosing. I married young and had two children. For seven years I spent my time at home pretending I was happy. I was far from happy and felt very trapped. I sank deeper and deeper into depression and became addicted to the antidepressants prescribed by my doctor. They blanked out what I was feeling—and the suicide attempts I experienced in my teens, resumed.

Death was when I would have it made. I decided the only way out of my marriage was to kill myself. Two weeks before Christmas I went to bed taking over a month's supply of antidepressants. It was the first time I felt hope in a long time—that death was my only hope. My suicide was unsuccessful and I woke up in intensive care two days later.

My children lived with my husband—I left and attended the day hospital for treatment but ended up for a month in a mental home. I got a part time job and joined AA and went into counselling. I was grieving for my lost childhood and I wanted it back. The trauma I had experienced over the years could have a two-fold effect. It could be the catalyst for creative change or the cause of self-destruction. I had done the self-destruction bit—I was now ready for the creative change.

I discovered whilst doing regression work that I spent nine months in my mother's womb being totally ignored by her. I felt my mother's reaction to her pregnancy such as ignoring me, hoping that I was a false alarm, and then anger towards me when she realised she was pregnant. Her reactions had a profound effect on my attitude not only towards her, but also towards how I felt about myself.

I had nine long months to marinate in all this negativity and shame that my mother felt towards her pregnancy. Her lack of recognition led me to feel unwanted, rejected and shamed. My birth scripts, which became life scripts, were,

I'm not wanted
I'm a mistake
I shouldn't be here, I don't belong.

During my delivery my mother refused to help me being born, and my terror of being suffocated and dying in the womb resulted in me having a profound sense of anger towards her for trying to kill me.

However, how was my mother to know that her own thoughts and feelings would have such a deep effect on me inside the womb? I myself was brought up with the knowledge that babies couldn't ever hear or see for weeks after being born, never mind being able to hear and feel inside the womb!

It was very emotional for me to learn that these maternal attitudes and feelings could leave a permanent mark on the unborn child's personality. I feel tremendous gratitude that I am able to connect the fractal patterns in my life from conception to the present time. I feel my compulsion to die through suicide came from the trauma I felt in the womb and the feelings I was marinated in; my mother's feelings and mine, became all confused; *I shouldn't be here, I'm a mistake,* and, *I'm going to die during this delivery.*

My way of attempting suicide through overdosing on medication can be connected to my mother taking medication for her migraine and blood pressure whilst pregnant with me. I was recreating time and time again through events in my life, my time in utero and birth trauma.

I feel certain that my mother's fear of death and dying came from being conceived herself after her sibling died at the age of six weeks. She would have been marinated in her own mother's feelings of grief, and her fear of perhaps losing her own baby.

By relating all of these fractals I am able to free myself from the destructive patterns at work in me. I can now differentiate what problems were mine and what problems were my parents.

How The Process Works

In experiential psychotherapy, regression is part of a process of diminishing one's defences against internal reality of pain and trauma. The stories we have included show how a person acts out their pre- and perinatal dynamics in gruesomely overt ways. There are suicidal tendencies, because the dynamics are so hidden, repressed and overlaid with defenses that the conscious mind has absolutely no access to, or insight into them being part of their unconscious dynamics.

The conscious mind is then completely able to convince itself that these dynamics are actual and real parts of the situation and therefore require an actual, real and extreme response. This can be brought about by a total dissociation from one's pre- and perinatal traumas but the trauma is internalised and self-inflicted. In this situation the suicide may be completed and death occurs.

When the total and complete dissociation of the pre- and perinatal trauma has not happened and it is much closer to the surface, although still not in consciousness, it is more likely to be allowed to emerge into consciousness, be relived, healed and then removed forever as a motivation to end one's life.

Conclusions & The Future

It may seem an incredible idea that people attempt suicide because something went wrong, either as far back as conception, or in utero, or with their birth process. Society is slow to recognise the importance of the primal period but the evidence of the power of imprinting from this time has increased dramatically over the last ten tears.

Preconception care and the physical health of the unborn is an area where more knowledge is being given to new parents to be. Prenatal education and classes for parents go back many years but there seems to be a gap in the care of pregnant women, probably more so in the Western world, than in the East where often the spirituality of a nation gives more energy to the developing baby.

The major sin of humanity may well be ignorance—and this is the lack of information on the area of pre- and perinatal influence on later suicide and other post traumatic stress syndromes.

Behind every death by suicide are hidden factors—and the inexperienced has to be experienced to find the circuit breakers, if this is possible with a client.

Maybe the sceptics are those who have never experienced the depth of human despair and the desire to die. Being sensitive to the awareness of the pain of the client, who is in the tenderest of places, where the original pain occurred, and to believe that the client is referring to experiences that actually happened, is a responsibility we owe to them.

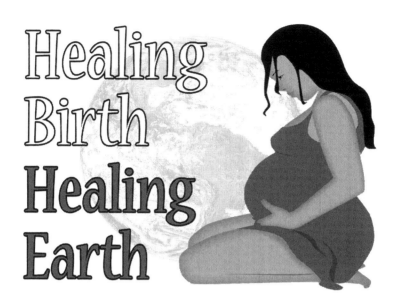

PART FOUR

Chapter 13

WIDER IMPLICATIONS

FRACTALS FROM THE WOMB

Fractals From The Womb

Think beginnings, and you are present at the birth of a child and the birth of our universe. Think middles, and you witness the child's growth to maturity, the movement of atoms and stars and planets and the evolution of life in its myriad forms. Think endings and you stand witness to death and our transitions to another form and the passing of old stars into new energies. Think connection and you know how it's all related—the cheese, the melody, the friend, the star, the starfish on the beach, the woman passing you in the street, the glint of dust floating in the sun's last ray; all part of a symphony of life in which part is part of each other and part of the whole and it is all one taste, one reality. ~ Jean Houston, *Awakening to Your life Purpose* 2011

During our lives I am sure there is always one teacher or mentor who touches our hearts, minds or soul, lights up our path and puts meaning into why we are here. Alongside Frank Lake and his work, Jean Houston and her gifted way of working helped widen my levels of consciousness, open up my inner life and widened my inner visionary capacity. I first met Jean in in Ireland in 1987 when 90 people attended her workshop on *Creativity and Intelligence*, put on by the teachers in Drogheda. Many did well for themselves in Ireland using their own human potential and Jean made a difference here.

In 1991 I met Jean again in Atlanta, Georgia when she was the keynote speaker at the International Conference for Prenatal and Perinatal Psychology. It was in her dynamic lecture, *Preparing the Foetus, Repairing the Earth* that Jean introduced the idea of fractals and over the last twenty years it has transformed my life and work.

Even from the age of four years old I remember looking at the sky, puzzled by stars and what was in space and beyond. I always wanted to find out as much as I could about humanity and the world. This often meant going beyond the limits and exploring the time and events before birth has been part of my entelechy in life. My work is constantly helping myself and others to fill in details from past experiences to complete the incomplete details of our present life. The brain and our consciousness already do this but this new and beautiful concept of fractals has been brought to us by means of computer-aided mathematics and has enabled the whole history of pre- and perinatal psychotherapy to come into perspective.

What Are Fractals?

The term *"Fractal"* was invented by Benoit Mandelbrot, an IBM computer systems researcher. The term describes the new geometry of shapes that form in the wake of dynamic systems. Each part of a fractal has the same statistical character as the whole. The mathematical formula behind this geometry creates an image of an endlessly repeating pattern, which is known as the Mandelbrot Set. Such an image would have been impossible without the use of computer aided mathematics and digital imagery. An example of a fractal image can be seen on the cover of this book. The resultant Mandelbrot set can be magnified forever without losing coherence. The shapes have infinite precision—and do exist in the natural world. They form an icon which embodies an important aspect of how the world and universe works, and have been described as the *Thumbprint of God*.

It appears that computer technology has revealed one of the greatest mysteries of our universe by giving us the word *"fractals"* to describe the phenomenon of rhythms and patterns that can be seen all around us. Furthermore, if we magnify the Mandelbrot Set a million times, even a billion times, it would eventually cover the universe. It is an image of Infinity. It could have been discovered anytime in history by adding and multiplying forever but that would be too complex for a human to compute. It was not until 1st March 1980 in New York that this concept was discovered, at the beginning of the era of new technology.

Fractal Patterns In The Natural World

Fractal patterns are far more than a complicated mathematical idea. They are repetitions of the same general patterns, even the same details, at both ascending and descending scales. They tell us that the universe and all that it contains is made up of folded realities within self-similar worlds. They have characteristics of self-similarity. Fractal patterns are all around us, above us and within us.

Trees are fractals, with their repeated patterns of large and small branches with similar details found even in the smallest twigs. Even a single leaf shows fractal repetitions of the whole tree in its shape and in the branching of its veins. In a broccoli or cauliflower you will find fractal geometry at its best, with florets arranged in self-similarity scales. Also for a total fractal experience, peel the leaves from an artichoke. The coastline of a country, or rocks and mountains also show fractal repetitions. The patterns of the weather; the turbulence in the wind; the rhythms pounded out by African drums and the landscapes of nature all embody fractals.

The existence of fractals in nature show us the holistic hidden order behind things, it reveals a harmony in which everything affects everything else, and above all, an endless variety of interwoven patterns. In the human body these endless, ever-replicating patterns are seen in the systems of the body—such as the circulatory system with branching vessels and the nervous system with branching neurons.

These patterns are mirrored in the wider universe. A spiral nebula in space, that measures hundreds of light years across, is based upon fractals. It looks remarkably similar to something that measures a thousandth of a centimeter, such as the eye of a firefly. One can be seen as the fractal resonance of the other—the resonance of the microcosm of the macrocosm.

Key Fractals

A fractal pattern, and one which is out of awareness almost certainly condemns us to play out the pattern again until it becomes conscious and understood. Here pre- and perinatal psychology, by bringing the primal origin into awareness is where the pattern may become changed. It can be changed or healed to the point of having little or no effect anymore in our lives. If the issue is still being attracted into our life experience, eg rejection—our reaction to the issue is changed.

The importance of parental health at the cellular level of ovum and sperm is crucial and advisable to provide the best possible beginning to new life. Globally we can no longer expect the health and development of the newborn to be left by chance by DNA and nature. The planet and nature are not exactly in a healthy state. How we live our lives affects the earth and lack of respect by us for our planet has affected our life force.

There are key fractals in the events and experiences of life. I am a fractal! You are a fractal! Our whole being is a Great Fractal. We are all made up of millions of fractals on an indeterminate number of levels all influenced by the environment. Each individual is made up of fractals right down to the single cell before it is fertilised by the sperm. Key fractals from before conception are the state of the energy of father and mother, and the dynamics and energy of the sperm and ovum. A tired sperm, a lively sperm, and excited sperm fusing with an exhausted ovum or a lively ovum—whatever the state of the parents will affect the receptive or unreceptive ovum and reflect upon the incoming new life.

Dr. Bruce Lipton

Lipton's work shows that everything within or without which can be considered the cellular environment affects its consciousness for good or bad depending in the stimulus received. Lipton has replaced the notion of nature and nurture with environment. This is an important aspect of pre- and perinatal work as the blastocyst, growing embryo and foetus experience the environment of the womb. The emergence of fractal patterns in the developing new life stems from the state of the parents at conception—and is a reality. We need to improve the generations that have gone before us in order to recreate healthier fractal waves to improve a better quality of life for as many people as possible. There is a wholeness involved in consciousness of who we are.

Fractals form a major part of us. Then how much more do we need to know whilst we are alive? We have a consciousness and intellect that can ask fundamental questions about our existence as well as the passion to uncover profound insights that govern each individual, the human race and our universe.

Making The Invisible, Visible

Our role may just be beginning and the discoveries in pre- and perinatal psychotherapy are only the tip of the iceberg. But it is a deep human desire to find out the workings ot the world and ourselves. Fractals were the hidden dimension before computer technology and human consciousness was not aware of them. It has made the invisible, visible and found order in chaos and disorder.

Fractals In Human Living

When I first heard Jean Houston lecture on Fractals in Atlanta in 1991 I knew I was hearing one of the most important aspects of my life and work as a researcher of foetal consciousness. At first I saw them as patterns and rhythms of life, keeping it simple for my students to understand. I am deeply grateful to Jean for giving me permission so generously to use her words and work in whatever ways I wish. This has freed me up to follow the concept of fractals in life and death itself from preconception onwards.

I gave a lecture on Fractals at the United Nations in Vienna around 1996 on *The Zodiac and Fractals*. The listeners were spellbound. As far as I know all my diagrams and notes are still in the UN library, as they were photographed and mounted to be kept for further use! During that lecture, a young man, a mathematician, stood up and asked if he could write out the mathematical equation of fractals on the flipchart. What he produced was the mathematical equation for infinity.

Again this changed my whole concept of life. Infinity—the depth and meaning of life as I had never conceived it before. We can live our lives simply looking at patterns, like a knitting pattern for example, but fractals is a very much deeper, more complicated pattern leading us into infinity. Fractals tell me that I am part of something that I never knew was believable. The older and wiser I grow, the more in touch I become with myself, other people, nature, understanding creativity and the cosmos. Fractals help me understand the interconnected world of patterns, rhythms, intertwined relationships, layer upon layer on concepts which form interconnectedness.

A few years ago I had to stop *growing* and give myself time and space because the depth of understanding being reached by fractal reality was more than my mind and body were able to comprehend and retain. It was like becoming the cosmos, universe, holding all knowledge—beyond what a human body, mind and spirit is meant to be whilst in a physical body. This is what the difference has been and is for me. Knowing that I have to keep grounded in my physical body but with the full realization that we are greater than this. I believe from conception we possess this great ability—and are part of something so much greater. We are part of the physical world but are very much more than that.

Our consciousness points us in the direction that there is much more to our own world than the physical that science describes. Something deep within, is this the spiritual being that has become physical? This incites us on to the idea of a divine mind or a divine purpose. Are we overcoming our fears and finding the energy connection to do what our Souls want us to do?

Do Our Souls Contain The Positive Fractal Patterns?

In November 1998 I wrote two short pieces of prose. In retrospect I did not see the fractal meaning at the time. It is hoping for understanding and the co-operation of the parents for future conception:-

The Soul Sent From Afar To The Parents-To-Be

I am a soul sent from God or from the Creator, whatever the Great Spirit is on your belief. I am a spiritual being sent to inhabit a physical body and to live a life upon planet earth. I ask for your love and care and attention that I may also love you, my parents, to treasure and respect the Earth upon which we shall walk together. If you love each other with genuine love and care for each other gently and respectfully—and the union of your love conceives me —I will be conceived in love and will walk all the days of my earthly life within that love.

Preparation By The Future Parents For Conception

The place that I come from is of peace, of stillness, sanctity and joy. It is a place of joy where all is harmony and beauty, where all may live in the light of healing and love. Deep in your soul you know this place, but life's difficulties have hidden your sacredness from you and your loved ones on earth. For my conception I ask you, for my sake, to be positive and loving and to prepare for my coming into being. I come from this place of beauty and this bliss, ecstasy, love and peace will stay with me if you are willing to prepare yourself before my conception.

It is children who ask questions about where they have come from and how they arrived on the planet. Their experience of birth and before birth is still not too far in the distant past. The adults in seeking truth about their existence ask the questions of what they are about and is there life after death? Looking ahead to what might be and speculating on the possibility of continuing consciousness for humanity. The question of whether consciousness continues into other states of life beyond has been a topic of study and thought almost to the beginning of humanity's existence.

At this point in our new millennium our consciousness turns to birth and death as people turn away from the many state established religions, or ways of life, to more contemporary forms of personal spirituality, shamanism, therapies, forms of meditation and visualisation, pilgrimages of walking—anything that will help us understand life and death. Often it seems that throughout the ages, death has been given more energy and time than birth! Yet now we have the knowledge and techniques to search the fractal links of our conception and birth to our lives and death. All of our lives can be seen as parts of the interpenetrating wave of the current time, psyche and memory. Jean Houston believes that the fractal waves of our lives are the stories rolling through our earlier and later lives. We may believe that their deeper currents, as in all lives, may be nothing more than the fractal waveforms of the Mind of the Maker, the Creator or Creative Spirit who started it all in the first place. Working as a psychotherapist I have to help people overcome the trauma of life in order to touch in with their creativity and human potential.

I believe the disorder, trauma and patterns happen before birth and so my entelechy is to help people become aware of the importance of the first nine months of life, in utero. This has an effect upon the rest of our lives on so many fractal levels. At some depth it appears to be something within reach that we are not able to grasp until we are ready—and that may well be at the end of our journey. I am that Fractal and everyone is their own Fractal depending on every single life experience that we have ever had. It makes us that very unique individual different from anyone else on the planet.

Fractals In Pre- and Perinatal Psychology

This concept of the fractal is both relevant and helpful in the understanding of pre- and perinatal psychology and psychotherapy. Frances Mott never lost sight of his idea of universal design, with patterns repeating endlessly throughout creation. This idea of endlessly repeating patterns of behaviour and belief, operating since conception has become central to our work at Amethyst. Let us speculate also that if we could look at the events in a human life in the same way as we look at branches of a tree, we might discover another order of fractals that recur in the happenings, moods, tragedies and comedies of human lives.

Pre-Conception And Conception

Putting the concept of fractals upon preconception and conception, we find that our life reflects the rhythm and pattern of the state of our parents and their lives, even before our conception. Frank Lake described early experiences as *patterns or principles of perceptual organization for later experiences* and serve as underlying prototypes for later complex reaction patterns. Fractals seem to be the descriptive link for Frank Lake's hypothesis that everything that happens in the birth trauma has already happened at conception and in the first trimester, the first three months of life.

At Amethyst we have continued to work on Lake's hypotheses. We often see, clearly demonstrated in the lives of our clients that the way parents prepare for the conception of their baby, their state of mind at the time of conception and the environmental situation are all reflected in the way they were are in utero and the type of birth that they experienced. In every life these repeating fractals colour the individual personality and lifestyle. It decides the jobs and careers we choose and even affects the way we die. The new physics has probed more deeply into the dimensions of energy and the forces of the moving universe that our world has more subtle realms of mind and consciousness. We are fractals, our blue planet is seen as a living organism, breathing and living as humanity.

We are interconnected and the earth responds energetically to the way it is treated by its inhabitants—us. Energy is connection and if that 'connection' is missing from conception the adult may have enormous difficulties in reaching out to others in relationships. Perhaps this may be the missing link in many people's lives. It brings to mind the wonderful painting of Michelangelo's on the ceiling of the Sistine Chapel in Rome. The hand of God reaching out to the hand of humanity, making that connection in *love*, is the example of the love connection necessary for the energy connection when conceiving a new human life.

Womb Trauma & Birth Trauma

The fractal resonances of conception trauma, womb trauma and birth trauma in turn impact on personality, characteristics, responses, attitudes, personality, relationships and careers, to name but a few.

We live our lives from the glory or trauma of our early beginnings. Severe damage caused in the intra-uterine period may cause almost irreparable damage to the growing embryo or foetus. This imprinting causes a fractal pattern, with patterns of irrational behaviour throughout childhood and adulthood that constantly repeat the original injury and the emotional consequences of it.

The work involves finding circuit breakers to change the negative patterns in many situations. We can, with appropriate help, re-pattern our lives to become positive human beings with a better quality of life.

Finding the keys to unblocking negative patterning, or freeing the positive fractals, is the way to find the integration necessary for moving forward in life and not carrying baggage that often is not ours, but belongs to mother of sometimes generations of the family. The recognition of the fractal, or the coding that has gone deep into our psyche, can change by bringing into consciousness the emotional feeling, the physical sensation and the historical memory of the primal trauma to heal the negative fractal of the present day.

A Positive Fractal

Life is full of fractals containing similar patterns and self-similarity! There are events and recurring patterns and coding which show critical keys to personality development and deeper purposes. Some may call it conditioning but I prefer to call it also learning development through positive experiences which may seem quite unimportant at the time. When I was three or four my parents used to take me to visit an aunt whose husband had died in the Second World War. He was my Uncle Bill and my aunt had many of his books that he had as a child. Some of these books were the *Wonder Book of Why And What, How Things Work, How Things Were Built*. Although I couldn't read all the words at this age they were fascinating books and I was always in a hurry to get back to my aunt's house to see what I could learn next!

It must have been these books that encouraged me to take apart a small grandfather clock that my grandmother lifted off the wall to clean! Then my father's gold watch that I removed from the drawer he kept it in, took it into the garden shed and proceeded to take it apart! I did get into trouble but I also knew the families were having a quiet laugh when they thought I was not listening! This laughter, amidst the trauma of the war taught me it was OK to be curious, to understand how things worked, what made me tick and also to go to the edge and find out whatever the answer was to the question, *Why?*

Primal Fractals

It is so encouraging to know that even Janov is also coming to the conclusion that we re-enact repeating patterns from the past. We just need the vocabulary to be able to talk about it. The fractal concept could well help heal the rift that appeared between Janov and the rest of the world in the 1970's—and that we all rejoice in the same revelation.

Present Life Fractals

You can track your own present day life themes backwards, into earlier life situations. You may find that some patterns may have begun in early childhood, but many of the deeper earlier traumas which positively and negatively affect your life will be found in the pre and perinatal period of life, shaped also by the influence of the environment of your mother's pregnancy during your nine-month period in the womb. It is also possible to track present day life themes backwards in your own life into ancestral lives. Many of them recur as waves, in different contexts, origin. In the future one may see these waves of similarity and chaos in character, personality and existential events repeating in one's physical and spiritual descendants throughout time. This is how fractals can make history, as we live out our fractals from the past. Frank Lake wrote:

The great danger is that, as many times before, we will interpret the fact of recession, on whatever scale or level it affects us personally, by evoking similar patterns of conflict and response from the past, that is, by regression. If this happens, it will be a regression, not to post-natal human levels of experience, but to pre-natal first and third trimester levels, of constrictions, threatening pressures and to similar patterns derived from even more crushingly frightening births.

Chapter 14

NARCISSISM: HUMANITY'S SECRET WEAPON OF MASS DESTRUCTION

Narcissism

It has taken some years for me to come to terms with the destructive narcissistic people in my own life, and the devastation caused to my own vulnerability and self-esteem. It was a major shock to realise how naively I had allowed this to happen, and to accept my lack of knowledge and understanding of narcissistic behaviour.

To look at it in another way is the lamb being led to the slaughter, in a silent and absorbing way by the perpetrator. This ignorance I have found not only in myself, but others, who in discussion, have completely overlooked the element of destructive narcissism and its devastating effect on victims, namely our clients and ourselves. It is a very powerful, silent way of destroying all of the good things around and creating energy of such negativity and destruction, that if not recognised and dealt with it does become a secret, unrecognised weapon of mass destruction in relationships, families, groups, companies, governments and countries.

Destructive narcissists have the ability to make everyone around them feel like needless idiots. A picture jumps to mind of Patricia Routledge playing the part of Mrs. Bucket, or as she prefers to be called *Mrs. Bouquet*, in the classic television programme *Keeping Up Appearances*. Her narcissistic approaches, sometimes overemphasised, dramatize her comically as the Queen Bee, with all life revolving around her. Her poor demented husband puts up with it all, is sucked dry by his wife, her demands, needs and attention-seeking behaviour. Although dramatized in a comedy, she is always right, but however hard he tries, he always gets it wrong. The writers have used comedy to illustrate narcissistic society, whether conscious or unconsciously—but speaking to husbands married to narcissistic wives their lives are far from easy and they may be living their lives in torment, unbeknown to colleagues and friends.

Destructive Narcissism

Destructive narcissism has presented itself to me in my work as a psychotherapist, encountering clients whose lives have been devastated by narcissistic mothers, fathers, brothers, sisters, spouses, partners, bosses and contacts who completely disempower the people around them, those under their authority, who have to suffer living or working with a control freak. Their demands often elicit protests and resistance, which in turn irritates the narcissist, who then becomes more stubborn and inflexible and the frustration and irritation in the relationship deepens. The disdain, rage and defiance towards the recipient are unbelievable, totally unexplainable and are all completely unacceptable, abusive behaviour.

It may only be a disagreement on who the best tennis player is in the world; if you don't agree with their choice the dramatics and hysteria may well be let loose! You must agree with them because they are never wrong! The problem has to be acknowledged before it can be addressed and because of this many narcissists remain undiagnosed. Unfortunately destructive narcissism has seriously overshadowed the characteristics of healthy narcissism so we do need to look at what both ends of the scale of narcissism exhibit. My understanding of healthy narcissism has clarified in the past years and encouraged me to help others to have a more positive attitude toward life and living.

Healthy Narcissism

Narcissism of varying degrees is in all of us. It is a term with a wide range of meanings. In healthy narcissism it is seen as high outward self confidence in line with reality. The healthy narcissist enjoys power, uses it wisely; as the last two Presidents of Ireland have shown. They have real concern for others and their ideas, and do not exploit or devalue others. They can have great leadership skills and are able to have vision and follow through with ideas. They are often skillful orators which make them charismatic: displaying personal magnetism and stirring enthusiasm amongst listeners.

Healthy narcissism is a required element within the normal development of an individual. It is the investment of energy in a real genuineness of understanding the Self. The accepted individual blooms into an emotionally rich, creative, productive adult. They are able to feel a full range of emotions, share in the emotional life of others, and pursue their abilities with real self-esteem and no self-doubt.

This is all founded on a healthy childhood with support for self-esteem, responsible behaviour and respect towards others. Healthy narcissistic world leaders when military, religious and political arenas dominated society were people like Napoleon Bonaparte, Mahatma Ghandi and Franklin D. Roosevelt. Social change brought individuals like Thomas Edison, Henry Ford and John D Rockefeller.

There are many narcissists at the helm of schools, businesses, organisations and governments who are highly effective people. The challenge to their colleagues is that they ensure their leaders do not self-destruct or lead the organisations into disaster.

It was George Bernard Shaw who said that some people see things as they are and ask why; narcissists see things that never were and ask why not? Into my mind jumps some of the greatest thinkers and great minds whose ideas have shaped modern civilisations.

Philosophers, scientists, artists like Aristotle, Plato, Galileo, Archimedes, Leo Tolstoy, William Shakespeare, Leonardo da Vinci, Sigmund Freud, Isaac Newton and Albert Einstein, who in 1999 was named by Time Magazine as *"Person of the Century"*. It was Einstein who reminded us we cannot solve problems from the same level of consciousness that created them.

We Need Visions

As psychotherapists we know that the consciousnesses that can find solutions to such problems in clients need models with matured possibilities. We need visions of what the possible human can be, using our healthy narcissism to go beyond academic excellence and use our skills as humanistic and integrative psychotherapists. Our work, though difficult at times, can be extremely exciting and rewarding in what Jean Houston calls the *re-genesis of society*. Jean herself is one of the foremost visionary thinkers and doers of our time, and one of the principal founders of the Human Potential Movement to which we all belong in our work as psychotherapists.

An Unrealistic Sense Of Superiority

Destructive narcissism is displayed with an unrealistic sense of superiority. Power is pursued at all costs, with no thought or feeling for others, and never any remorse or shame for wrongdoing or exploitation. There is a lack of values; the individual is easily bored and restless. The foundations for this are seen as no true sense of self and no consideration for other people, with boundaries being non-existent. The most obvious observation of narcissism is of the perpetrator of sexual abuse but recognition of narcissism in other forms of abusive, yet subtle behaviour, is required by the therapist.

According to the American Psychiatric Association (1994) the Narcissistic Personality Disorder is diagnosed by individuals showing five or more of the following symptoms:-

Self-importance; exaggerating achievements and talents.
Preoccupied with fantasies of unlimited success, power and ideal love
Believes they are special and unique; only associate with status people
Requires excessive admiration
Has strong sense of entitlement towards favourable treatment
Is exploitive of others, takes advantage to meet own ends
Lacks empathy and is unwilling to recognise needs of others
Is often envious of others
Regularly shows arrogant, haughty behaviours or attitudes

The Destructive Narcissist In Relationship

As the narcissist continues to make demands, the recipient of such behaviour may walk away, realising that the effort is too much to deal with. It takes a lot of energy to live with such demands. There may be such loyalty that the recipient stays in the relationship, but is clearly lacking in knowledge of what is really going on, and even if they do, having no idea how to deal with it. Questioning the behaviour, wondering what is wrong with the person, or what is going on in the situation may well remain unsolved unless the different stages of narcissism are brought into consciousness and understood.

The narcissist seems quite unaffected and continues to wear down anyone who would even dare to think or feel differently from themselves. People are their property and they truly believe they own the people closest to them. They may seduce someone with low esteem by pretending to love them or by offering them money. Any inclination to decline or to behave differently is interpreted by the narcissist as betrayal.

The attitudes and behaviour exhibited by narcissists can stir up many different kinds of feelings in the people whose lives they are intertwined with. They seem to find your weakest point—or you respond from your weakest point, maybe personal rejection, lack of confidence or lack of self-esteem, or just being too *'nice'*, which leads you into a sometimes intolerable situation.

When you interact or try to relate with narcissists, their distortions of reality can push you into questioning your own truth, and doubting your own perceptions—and so narcissism is not recognised. When you walk into a room where they are, they may be absolutely silent, waiting for the visitor to ask how they are. They are not interested in anyone else, just for you to know their opinions and thoughts. If you leave the room, they may follow you to make sure you do not speak to anyone else and they have your full attention. Are you, the reader, beginning to recognise this cycle in your life, relationships, and situations or with clients who need help?

The recipient of this type of behaviour can be stressed to breaking point. If the narcissistic behaviour continues it may lead to abusive relationships, bullying, cruelty, suicide and God forbid, murder.

Narcissism must be faced and dealt with—either by the victims or the perpetrator. It is more likely to be the victims, as the narcissist is always right and rarely would last in a therapy room as they would regard the therapist as below them, completely on the wrong track and, in fact, they know better than the therapist. Psychotherapists have a responsibility to understand the nature of narcissism and recognise the effects of it on their clients who come into the therapy room broken, devastated and often lost.

How Does A Healthy Narcissist Become A Destructive One?

I am not sure that many healthy narcissists do become destructive ones. With my research in the pre- and perinatal area I understand that we are born with positive or negative tendencies according to our experiences in utero; research is on-going in this area. Frank Lake once wrote that adults carry mother's negativity from utero for life, unless the key to unlocking it in the pre-and perinatal period is found. Negative umbilical affect or the maternal foetal distress syndrome that clients relive in regression work is evidence that the pain carried was never ours in the first place. We were marinated in it in our very first environment in the womb.

It is also important to recognise that healthy narcissists are sensitive to criticism because they are extraordinarily sensitive. They are not thick-skinned and bruise easily. Criticism threatens their self-image and confidence of vision. This has a major consequence of the difficulty of not listening to criticism particularly when they feel threatened or attacked. I can see how healthy narcissists can become destructive when people in life have misunderstood their intentions to wanting to do well, or being inventive and energise ideas. They need the support of understanding people around them, to give them the affirmation they need. Otherwise, under extreme distress they can deteriorate into paranoia, and this is when the healthy narcissists can fall into destructive narcissism.

It is important for the therapist to note that the Narcissistic Personality Disorder is usually diagnosed by a trained mental health professional like a psychologist or psychiatrist as many therapists are not trained or well equipped to make psychological diagnoses.

Origins Of Narcissism

Psychoanalysts and psychologists believe that the foundation for full-blown narcissism is established right after birth, continuing through the formative years up to the age of 5 or 6. They see the 'terrible twos' as the time when youngsters go through the self-centred stage and are excruciatingly demanding, as part of the developing narcissistic spectrum firstly known as primary narcissism.

Adult narcissists tend to display these immature, childish tendencies, of lack of empathy for others; sadistic streaks; a cruel immature sense of humour; and destructive tendencies to unwitting people. A two year old's world revolves around them. They are the most important person in the world, parents and everyone else tends to their needs. If this does happen and the child does not learn that people will not always satisfy their needs—and parents continue to satisfy their every whim—then the narcissism develops.

The adult faced with the pressures of life, family, career and social intervention, implodes psychologically and regresses back to the early negative childhood patterns of behaviour. The healthy human being learns to live with life's disappointments, accepting the downside and traumas as part of life, but this is not so with narcissists who may also continually complain about everything not going their way. Alexander Lowen wrote in 1985:

Deprivation seems to affect the emotional development of a child in much the same way as horror does. Both conflict with the individual's inborn sense of the natural order of things. Both deprivation and horror have an element of unreality making them incomprehensible to the individual.

So what is seen here is when the child's sense of reality is upset, the child struggles to re-establish the expected environment. If this is not achieved the individual detaches emotionally, lives in an unreal inner world, develops a false self with no idea who they really are, and becomes on the way to developing secondary narcissism, and with no help, eventually the Narcissistic Personality Disorder.

Pre- And Perinatal Origins of Narcissism

My research in pre- and perinatal psychotherapy and foetal consciousness has led me to believe the origins lay further back than childhood. Of course, it may be fed into the childhood trauma as I mentioned in the last section, where the fractal wave or imprinting of these early fractals or patterns keep repeating and become part of the evolving development of the individual. I believe the onset of pathological narcissism lies in abuse in infancy and before birth to the unborn baby. This may be inflicted unwittingly by parents, medical professionals and authority figures in the life of the foetus in the womb.

The development of the true identity of each unique individual begins at conception. Here begins the sensations and dynamics of physical, emotional and environmental experiences which influence the real identity of the new personality. Any unloving situation in that first blast of conception energy may be experienced from forced sexual activity, rape, anger or drunkenness and they all become part of the deprivation pattern of need.

In utero, the foetus may experience alcohol, smoking, forced sex during pregnancy, amniocentesis, external harm from domestic violence and parental arguments—anything that shatters or cuts the nurturing from mother and the foetus has the horrific experience of being isolated and having no nurturing from the very beginning. Deprivation within the womb can be life threatening—and the unborn baby may fight and struggle for survival. The sense of aloneness and loss of contact with mother terrifies the baby. After continuous struggles for the baby to contact the mother without success; the reality of the desire for intimacy and closeness; of needs not being met; of no-one being there for the vulnerable, fragile foetus.

This tiny being accepts it. The intra-uterine trauma that was so devastating killed the tiny person emotionally. The pain never leaves and the individual creates a protective barrier that is insulation from the external world of people. The reality becomes a false self with no understanding of the real self. The foundations for narcissism and the borderline personality have been laid, even before birth.

Pathological narcissism is a defence mechanism intended to deflect hurt and trauma from the victims *'true self'*, their entelechy, and the person they are meant to become, into a *'false self'* which is omnipotent, invulnerable and omniscient. The adult finding themselves in this terrible conflicting and opposing state of mind becomes the type of person that others fear and avoid. The victim may become completely seduced by the omnipotent bully.

Loss Of A Monozygotic Twin In The Womb

Althea Hayton, a private researcher exploring the psychological effects on the surviving twin of the death of a co-twin before birth, has put forward the hypothesis that narcissism may be the result of being a surviving identical twin. Research carried out in the USA has shown that one in eight people is a womb twin survivor, they lost a twin before birth and many mothers are unaware in many instances that they were carrying twins as this happens at the zygote or embryonic stage. Medically, one zygote splits to create two embryos and one sucks the life out of the other. This is the twin-twin transfusion, where when one twin dies the blood of the dead twin may pass into the body of the survivor via the shared placenta. Metaphorically speaking Althea explained that the blood of the twin who didn't make it, had it sucked out by the survivor, and so is set up the imprint of living like a leech on other people, feeding off their weaknesses in order to survive themselves.

The Stages of Narcissism

Almost everyone is narcissistic to some degree, ranging from one end of the scale to another, and it may be difficult recognising the degree of narcissism to be dealt with. The term narcissism was chosen by Sigmund Freud, from the Greek Myth of Narcissus, whose fate was to fall in love with his own reflection in a pool of water. Unfortunately the negative side of narcissism is seen generally, and is a very narrow-minded view often seen as self-love, without the devastating effects it can cause in relationships. The narcissist we recognise as unhealthy is someone who, no matter what age, has not yet developed emotionally or morally owing to the negative childhood or infancy experiences mentioned in the origins of narcissism. When it becomes a psychological condition it may be defined as a total obsession of self, to the exclusion of almost all other interactions with people. These behaviours and attitudes become defence mechanisms to protect an underdeveloped self at the expense of the feelings of other people and may develop into the Narcissistic Personality Disorder.

There is a duality in narcissism ranging from the exterior in which a mask is worn and the character traits are self-admiration, self-centeredness and self-regard and manifest as severe selfishness and disregard for the needs and feelings of others. The excessive need for admiration and affirmation may be present to such an extent that it severely damages an individual's ability to live a happy and productive life. In contrast the narcissist may appear very defensive. The individual may become extremely introverted in social situations, tending to avoid deep commitments to family or work. They live off all who surround them but this all covers a deep fragility they hardly dare face. An effective or other way of understanding narcissism is in pain. To work with any stage of unhealthy narcissism the therapist needs an empathic and compassionate way of understanding it.

Working With The Recipients

To work with survivors of narcissistic mothering, fathering, siblings or partners, the therapist needs a patient and delicate way of explaining to the client the real effects of the narcissistic person in their lives, who has been cruel, spiteful, heartless, sadistic and grievously unloving to them in their lives. It is a painful, agonising affliction to be told that you had a narcissistic mother or person in your life, when you have loved them unconditionally without realising the damage that has been done to you. It takes a long time for this to be absorbed by the client and this is where the real patience of the therapist is tested.

Narcissistic Traits In The Therapy Room

Recognising and unravelling confusion and conflict in personal relationships, with underlying negative, narcissistic trends, is the job of the therapist! There are three major themes that arise in the therapy room, firstly the recognising and owning of personal narcissism by the therapist, whether healthy or negative; secondly the narcissistic client; thirdly, the client who is in need of healing, having been influenced by narcissists in their lives and the devastation it has caused them.

Narcissism In The Therapist

Therapists need to recognise and own their own personal experience, with healthy or negative narcissism, in their own personality and its effect upon all aspects of their lives and clients. The therapist does have power in the therapy room and integrity is needed to acknowledge the reactions and responses by the client projecting the authority figure onto them, and the reaction and responses by the therapist themselves. Therapists know that a narcissist's striving for power stems from a deep sense of humiliation suffered as a child. If a power struggle emerges between a therapist and client then it is imperative for the therapist to reflect on their own degree of narcissism, as any supervisor would recommend. In fact wherever power struggles emerge in life in relationships, families, groups, committees, organisations and businesses it seems this is a useful reflection for healing.

There are narcissistic snares within a psychotherapist's career which show themselves as personal, unrealistic expectations and aspirations for caregiving. One is falling under the narcissistic snare of omnipotence, heal all, know all and love all. It is an unrealistic, but understandable aspiration, in which the less experienced therapist may land up in trouble by taking on clients whose problems are well beyond their experience. Intuition and empathy are in a therapist's point of reference but need to be used wisely with where the reality is, and not where the therapist thinks the client is.

The Narcissistic Client

The therapist has to be very strong and have the strength of personality to survive narcissistic clients. As they operate from a dominating place they cause emotional temperatures to rise, promote people into angry responses and have an underlying need to destroy everything. Although they desperately need help, the resistance to change, or belief in anyone else's ideas but their own, is a hard nut to crack. Remember that no *'ordinary'* person will accept the narcissist with their delusions and they recoil immediately from the scene.

Narcissistic clients' comments may be related to the fact that therapy won't work. If they last a few sessions, some having done the rounds of the therapies, each session may be referred to as a waste of time, nothing is happening, nothing has changed.

The expectation is for the therapist to heal the client's negativity (which I personally believe comes from the negative umbilical effect in utero from mother), to tell them where the negativity comes from, guess what is wrong with them and if you don't, they project a strong sense of failure onto the therapist. Don't take it personally!

Failure Of Empathy

A major theme from the narcissistic client is their accusation, direct or indirect, of the therapist lacking understanding of what is going on for them. With their belief that psychotherapy isn't working, they may try to sabotage the therapist. This failure of empathy, as perceived by the client with their distorted vision, can permanently destroy the empathy from the therapist, a vital therapeutic tool to help the client resolve their deeper feelings of inadequacy. This destructive force may leave the truly empathic therapist totally drained of energy.

The Way Forward

The client may choose to leave the therapeutic relationship or stay in it to transform their lives. Whatever the decision, the therapist needs to see the weak, vulnerable little person inside and learn a strategy to deal with it. There are amazing life lessons to learn together, as long as the therapist remains strong for the client and also realise they are in a much stronger position than the client.

The client's behaviour may be destructive and terrifying but the vulnerable child is lost somewhere inside, in insurmountable pain. Clients presenting as typical borderline narcissists look normal on the surface. Superficially they look normal, and inside have very little feeling. They may acknowledge from an early age not being present to anyone or anything. Something traumatic happened to them very early on, to turn a human being into being non-feeling, emotionally dead and resistant.

A way forward is the therapist pointing out the aspects of reality which is being denied, devalued or avoided. The client's vulnerability needs to be acknowledged at all times and no confrontation about behaviour which is destructive ever attempted. This would re-stimulate the trauma, resulting in the client not working out the answer to the problem themselves and getting insight—but resistance and transference acting out.

Complex interactions have taken place in the client's life depriving them of finding their real self. Therapists have their own limitations in unravelling the mysteries of negative, destructive narcissism, either in the narcissistic client or those damaged by narcissists.

The therapist may help, as in so many other client problems, in differentiating between the True Self and the False Self. Giving client time to draw comparisons and understand what they are working with may begin the healing.

The true self is the core of our being, the original 'you', unshaped or unconditioned by environment, upbringing or society. This is the state we were in at our conception and still exists. The true self is strongly guarded or hidden by the false self and patience is needed to reach it. The false self is that which has hidden and changed our real being. Our original personality and behaviour, there from our beginnings, have been altered.

Feelings become repressed, behaviour adapted to fit in with other's needs, particularly mothers, all done unconsciously.

We now know that babies are conscious in the womb, that babies sense their mother's needs and their own behaviour is adapted to respond to what mother needs. It creates the beginnings of the false self from a very early age. Further work will need a well organised way of working with the narcissism and be tightly supervised.

Clients Whose Lives Have Been Devastated By Narcissists

This third issue is the one mainly having to be dealt with by therapists and it can be a subtle issue to recognise amongst all the complications of a client's life. It could well be the dominating feature if picked up by a discerning therapist. It is the therapist's job to discover how verbal and non-verbal messages to the client from narcissists have translated into overachievement, feelings of self-criticism and self-sabotage. Feelings of lack of success may be due to no affirmations whatsoever from the people they most wanted it from during their self-development.

The main people who come into therapy are, unsurprisingly, daughters of narcissistic mothers, husbands of narcissistic wives, sons of narcissistic parents—whose expectations of their sons is intolerable, whether conscious or unconscious. Partners are often freer to leave the relationship if narcissism occurs in the relationship whether it is recognised or not, but often it is interpreted as bullying.

I am not sure that humanity really understands what the long-term consequences are on children who have been moulded by narcissistic parents. Usually this happens when it is in the best interest of the parents, and not their siblings. This type of parental love is certainly not unconditional. It is important to recognise that a natural defence against the narcissistic place is *double orientation* which is a form of dissociation which attempts to conceal a situation and go on acting as though it never happened. A good pointer for therapists working with these client difficulties.

Healing The Daughters Of Narcissistic Mothers

Due to the vastness of this subject I am limiting case studies by looking at a few comments from the therapy room from daughters of narcissistic mothers, although similar themes are present in other narcissistic relationships. The pain caused to the offspring of a narcissistic mother may be excruciatingly painful.

Born to a narcissistic mother means she always puts herself first, whatever has happened whilst she was pregnant, self may always have been first. The birth of the baby takes the attention away from her. Mother continues to put herself first and there will be no mother and baby bonding—ever. Relating to Dr. Frank Lake's Dynamic Life Cycle where acceptance is needed to achieve, the child or adult tries throughout life to please mother, with no success. The fractal or repeating pattern cripples the personality of the child or adult who can never understand the lack of recognition by mother, with no affirmations, no good comments. Looking after mother and her constant needs; listening to her constantly talking about herself and doing only what she wants to do and nothing else is an exhausting life style for adult survivors.

Nora, a 53 year old single survivor said:

Growing up I knew something was very wrong. There was no connection between Mam and myself. I tried to 'fit in' with what she wanted but it was never right for her. For example if we were getting ready to go to town to shop (and I would be in my 30's at this time) if the phone rang and I spoke to a friend for a few minutes, when I was ready mam decided she wasn't going after all. It took me years to realise she always wanted to be the centre of attention. Any distractions and she played up, blaming me for not considering her needs. She would never go anywhere that my poor father wanted to go, he couldn't do anything right.

Siobhan aged 47, another survivor, said:

It didn't matter what age I was, when I was around, her need of me was paramount. I had to do everything she wanted me to do. I fell completely into the trap, thinking I was a caring daughter and did what she wanted.

I had no mind of my own. When she wanted something from Da or me, and neither of us responded, sometimes from exhaustion, her cruelty was displayed by being silent and moody for days on end.

Breda, at 45 wrote:-
I came to resent her words, "If I were you…." They were completely and utterly controlling. If I stood up for myself telling her she was not me—back would come some demeaning remark insinuating that I was not capable of doing anything right. I was constantly bullied and battered emotionally.

Mary, at 29 years of age, wrote from the USA:
I became rebellious in my teen, not coping with Ma's expectations of me becoming who I wasn't. Curls, frills, dresses, even at six, seven and eight adorned me. I'd come back with torn skirts, ripped tops, and shredded blouses from climbing trees. I'd get really walloped and screamed at and my brother laughed. I wanted shorts and tops not frills and lace to play in. I know that my Ma lived her life through me. I couldn't fulfil her goals so I left the country at 19. She never forgave me, or wanted to speak to me again as it wasn't what she wanted.

Katie, in her 40's said:
I have had so many failed relationships and I am not married. I see now that it is because none of my partners have given me what I lacked as a child. It feels like the love I didn't get from my narcissistic mother will never be healed. I go overboard caring for everyone. I have to recognise too the narcissistic traits acquired from Mam, and now check why I do so much caring. It doesn't help me feel good.

Jackie, in her 50's wrote:-
After I had done some serious therapy sessions on my own low self esteem and lack of confidence I received a letter from a long term friend. I had never seen such a vicious, accusing letter and it hurt me deeply. In it she accused me of not knowing the first thing about being a Christian, of always being right, of spending money like water and to think before I opened my mouth as I was an awful person. I realised that over the months I had stood up for myself to heavy criticism from her and she didn't like it. She could not control me anymore and the therapy helped me stand up for myself. It was with shock that I realised I had been seduced for many years by a narcissistic personality who only put her own needs and emotion to the fore. I realised she had done this to many people around her but because of my own needs and the

influence of a narcissistic mother I had been completely duped by her. She was an emotional vampire who sneered at my suggestions and good works; she was out to nurture her own needs, lick her own wounds and undermine me the whole of our relationship. I severed the relationship as I was better being out of this dangerous and damaging situation. I could have sued her for what she was saying to other people about me, but I left it wisely, I believe. I did not want to be drawn into anger with her or rescind my appropriate assertions. I never saw her again.

The pain experienced by these clients is obvious. Mothers who are narcissistic are basically emotionally cold and exploitive. Ignoring their child's separation needs usually because they are totally ignorant of them. They mould their children into objects that fit their own emotional need of perfection.

David Winnicott wrote in 1965 that *as separation occurs, the mother who is not good enough is not able to implement the infant's omnipotence and so repeatedly fails to meet the infant's gesture, substituting her own, which is to be given sense by the compliance on the part of the infant, is the earliest stage of the false self and belongs to the mother's inability to sense her infant's needs.*

It is not rare for the children of narcissistic mothers to be the good child, they stay quiet, do not argue, do what they are told to do, are no trouble, toe the line and do not complain. Work on the false self and finding the true self can be worked side by side with healing the wounded child and infant.

Encouraging Healthy Narcissism

We are trying to teach people to understand healthy narcissism. I believe that to heal one person is to help to heal the world; it is our responsibility to transform negativity from many levels into positive, healthy narcissism for our children's children. If no recognition is given as to the power of devastation in destructive narcissism, it really is humanity's secret weapon of mass destruction. It can be transformed to become the most positive talent we have in the world to transform lives positively.

Chapter 15

THE HUMAN CHAKRAS

The Human Chakras

I believe, as many others do, that chakras—the human energy field of each human being—mirror the energy fields of the planet earth and that of the universe, in a similar way to fractals. These two ideas are closely linked and have been found useful when working with pre- and perinatal material.

The Chakras are the energy centres that make up the human energy field. These energies in the body not yet recognised by many in the Western world who believe there is no scientific proof of its existence. Certainly it would not be recognised by many working in traditional orthodox medicine, and those who have experienced it tend to be working now in their own therapeutic practices alongside one or two complementary therapies.

However, with the arrival over the past twenty years of Complementary Medicines and therapies which base their whole model on the presence of a human energy field, it is time to ponder over a whole new way of thinking and to ask what is happening in the field of Humanistic and Integrative Psychotherapy.

I believe there is a place for the use of the Chakras in Psychotherapy and the understanding of energy healing, which in some intangible way is already what many psychotherapists are doing —and what many clients want in our new millennium.

A Personal Perspective

I was introduced to the whole concept of the Chakras in 1981 when Rosalyn Bruyere first came to Ireland to teach her workshops on healing. I found the concept challenging, yet so simple to follow, and it gave me the insight and the answer to what I was looking for in my own healing, and also further integration of human understanding and the depth work with clients in my psychotherapeutic practice.

My excitement rose at the idea of being able to explore different levels of healing, not only psychologically, but in the whole sphere of body, mind, emotional and spiritual healing. I developed a significant understanding of the chakras in my own life, which helped my own energy levels, not only in experiencing the depth or frequency in which a trauma had *'gone in'*, but how energy patterns were changed on re-experiencing a trauma, bringing it back into consciousness and allowing it to dissipate. It made so much sense in so many areas of human trauma. I had also looked for a concept that could help me integrate rhythms and patterns of people's lives from conception to death, and I found answers in the concept of Fractal Patterns.

During these years the work of Jean Houston influenced me greatly and her writings sang of the integration of life events and her concepts of sacred psychology. In the fusing of secular psychology, psychotherapy and sacred psychology I found many answers. The chakras brought an understanding of the spiritual dimension. It was wonderful to recognise that it was not only the psychological level that I needed to work with but by experiencing my life in the seven major energy areas I could expand and contract in life according to the environment and situations I found myself in and not continually be in contraction as is the script of the forceps delivered birth such as my own!

Never was it more clear to me, in retrospect, as a young novice in religious life I was *'forced'* or expected to be spiritual, know how to pray—or have a healthy spiritual life (in the fourth, fifth, sixth and seventh chakras) when my basic needs for survival and relationships (in the first, second and third chakras) were so messed up in these three counselling chakras, as I call them, that I didn't know whether I was standing on my head or my heels! In my 20's I was trying to be spiritual at a deep level before I came to terms with being human.

I wonder how many more of us have found ourselves in this predicament. Not grounding the energy field can turn us into what I would describe as *'space cadets'* and I leave you to visualise what this means! Jean Houston wrote in 1996:-

In sacred psychology we take it for granted that our existential life is the largest part of our existence, while psyche is some anomalous misty stuff that we relegate to the basement. In sacred psychology however, we discover that it is not psyche that exists in us, but we who exist in psyche, just as the larger life of psyche exists in the realm of God.

Humanistic and Integrative Psychotherapy is not only looking at purely psychological problems of humanity. It helps each person to alleviate problems at many levels. This is for each individual to maintain a strong energy system capable of meeting the challenges of a constantly changing planet and evolving consciousness.

The integration of understanding energy into psychotherapy introduces the transpersonal element. In my own work as a trainer and psychotherapist, by introducing the use of chakras and understanding of the human energy field it has helped students and clients to find an equality of awareness, a humbling recognition of our humanness at all levels, in all dimensions, on many spheres. It opens up a wonderful dimension on a fractal level of the magnificent creativity of our spirituality and by this I am not speaking of religion.

As spiritual beings coming to terms with a physical body—the chakras appear to map the progress of personal consciousness from conception, the life of the embryo, to the higher stages of self-realisation and ultimate reunion with a Divine Source, whatever that might mean for individuals.

The Thoughts Of Other Writers

In antiquity the words *Know Thyself* written above the door of the temple in Delphi, Greece, had more than a decorative significance. The late Dr. John Rowan, in a presentation in March 1992 spoke of his translation of Ken Wilber's work and explained that we reach a more enlightened spiritual deepening within ourselves by experiencing the various therapies evolving today. The spiritual may be reached by knowing ourselves.

Chakras are part of Eastern Psychology and Philosophy, particularly introduced into the West through the tradition and practice of Yoga. Ken Wilber in his essay *Are the Chakras Real?* points out that awareness is not mandatory in the journey to liberation but physiological changes in the body associated with opening up the chakras in Kundalini Yoga can be viewed either as a cause or effect of changes in consciousness.

Rowan said that Jung never really understood or embraced Yoga and refused to talk about the top two chakras. Rowan also writes of the human potential to access levels of consciousness, and although deliberately changing some of the traditional naming of parts to fit a transpersonal model—he acknowledges that this is not far from the chakra system in yoga.

For psychotherapists still trying to make sense of people's problems through ordinary psychology the understanding of chakras may be very difficult. This also applies to those living in a social context which is unsympathetic to a change in thinking. Clients do move into the transpersonal area and psychotherapists in the western world need knowledge of the chakra system in order to understand cultural differences. Also to assist their clients in what might become spiritual emergencies according to Stan Grof, particularly when personal transformation becomes a crisis.

A Changing Way of Thinking

Traditionally, most of us when thinking of the mind, immediately think of the brain. Over the years, science has begun to postulate that the mind is not in the brain. Penfield wrote in 1976 that thought and memory seem to exist throughout the body; in 1948 Reich believed memory was being logged primarily within the body's fascia or connective tissues. In this respect Bruyere wrote in 1989 believes thought can also be described as a form of energy. Rupert Sheldrake favours the hypothesis that brains are like tuning devices and that the storage of memory is outside the brain and body.

Western society for many hundreds of years lost touch with the principles, harmony and unity known and expressed by many ancient cultures. The concept that we are all energy, pain is blocked energy and the mind is in the energy field around and through the body, and may or may not be controlled by the brain—has been literally unthinkable!

The Chakra system is at least a 5,000 year old way to integrate body, mind, emotions and spirit. If the mind is in the energy field, and the Chakra system is the human energy field—there is a valid reason for psychotherapists to study and understand it. From antiquity there have been various descriptions of the field of energy which emanates from the physical body. This luminous radiation was called an aura by the ancients. They knew a person's aura was a reflection of the soul—also reflecting much of the person's physical being. They also knew that these subtle energy fields generated that auric light.

Antiquity is filled with descriptions of spinning wheels of colour, subtle bodies of light within a denser larger human body. To a person who can see the auric field the chakras appear as little cyclones or whirling vortexes of energy. The words *aura* and *auric light* may send warning bells to some—because it rings of clairvoyance, spiritualism and matters that traditional Christians avoid. This mind set needs to be worked through and a changing way of thinking experienced. Chakras can be utilised in psychotherapy in a most acceptable way.

Scientific Proof

We know that all living matter radiates energy. Isaac Newton alluded to electromagnetic light as early as 1759. In the last twenty five years science is confirming the existence of the human energy field and the subtle energies generated from it.

In seven years of research at UCLA, Dr. Valerie Hunt was able to discuss the nature of Newton's electromagnetic light, which is called an electromagnetic field by today's scientists. In 1979 Dr. Hunt and Rosalyn Bruyere worked together on what came to be known as The Rolf Study which not only provided evidence that chakra energies or frequencies exist but also that they are connected in a very real way to our sensations, feelings and thoughts.

This highly thought of chakra system is a cornerstone of modern medicine and psychiatry in most oriental countries and is taught as a *'hard science'* in many Asian medical schools. Like so many aspects of 'new technology' today, chakras are beyond our perception but we know they are there! For example evidence of energy waves—they are scientifically proven through the waves from one mobile phone to another; also from a computer thousands of miles away your computer can receive an email that has travelled in a way that is unseen by our human eyes. This is the same as your energy field.

The Chakras are there—spinning wheels, discs of light, holders of information; spinning wheels of energy spinning in clockwise direction on the front of the body, and anti-clockwise on the back. Each chakra is a centre of activity dictating a particular attitude towards reality; transmitting, receiving, processing and integrating energy on an amplitude or frequency through every cell or fibre of your body. Impulses of energy carrying the information to transmit instructions for it to grow new cells, replicate, heal and continue all bodily functions, many of which we are not consciously aware of.

Ken Wilber wrote over twenty five years ago, that the chakras are part of Eastern psychology, but he emphasized that it is generally agreed by Eastern and Western psychology alike that the lowest levels of development involve simple biological functions and processes. This means that the lowest levels involve somatic processes, instincts, simple sensations and perceptions and emotional-sexual impulses.

The Chakras - Human Computer Discs!

When working with the chakras, mostly it revolves round the nature and function of seven primary chakras. There are actually over one hundred chakras in the body, found at each joint and also where every place a bone and nerve exists.

Each chakra has a personality with positive lessons and negative distortions. When, during human development the chakras have been distorted, these are the centres to work with in psychotherapy depending on the trauma and problems presented.

In my own practice over the years I have worked on the premise that the mind is in the energy field. Therefore, recall of past events is not only in the body cells which renew themselves frequently, but in the energy field. Unless the key is found and healing takes place, negative life patterns continue to be present in newly-formed cells.

This really does shine a new light onto how we all function. In some cases, the amplitude or frequency at which a trauma occurred needs to be reached during psychotherapy to allow a DC (Direct Current) Shift to happen.

This is particularly noticeable when a client is in shock and this could be a lifelong shock relating to childhood trauma, birth trauma or even before birth.

At this point it is important to realise that understanding and integrating the chakra system into psychotherapy is not to present an other-worldly discipline, borrowed from the cultures of the East, but an integration or blending of concepts from East and West.

The Three Lower Chakras

The three lower chakras are the counselling chakras. They lie over a major part of the excretory organs, from where clients need to excrete negativity from their lives. The first three chakras relate to the physical, emotional and intellectual aspects of life.

These three chakras are the ones that psychotherapists are dealing with, consciously or unconsciously with clients, for changing life patterns, and possibly before any transpersonal work is reached.

Physical illness often accompanies many of the psychological problems that clients present. Also when the physical body itself begins to go out of balance it sends signals that are not as easy to ignore as the psychological ones. In society today anaesthetising the psychological symptoms is prevalent—alcohol use drowns the sorrows and distresses of a life; prescribed drugs and others, numb out the negative emotions; smoking *'fogs up'* the energy field. Smokers may well not like their own energy field but may not be aware of this factor when coming into therapy.

Work in these lower chakras is vital, as so many illnesses, diseases and depression have their roots in the lower energies.The psychotherapist is aware of these factors but speaking of the damage that can be done to the mind of the client, may help a client to begin a physical activity that will stimulate the neurotransmitters and begin to help clear the energy field of *'smog'* and gently help the memories, feelings, words and events to be remembered.

The First Chakra

The red energy of the first, physical chakra, is where people need to take their power and understand and feel their sexual drive and energy. It is the source of everything we sense about physical reality, is known as the physical body and is the centre of our vitality. It contains our own sense of ourselves. All survival needs and self-preservation instincts are related to this centre. If there is an imbalance in this physical chakra it can put all the energies of the other chakras out of balance, so it is of vital importance to balance this chakra. The age of the chakra is four years old, and at this age the child understands self to be separate from others.

The one thing in life that is yours, and belongs to no-one else, is your body. It is possible to tell the personality of a person and from out of which chakra they may be living their lives. Many famous men and women throughout history could be called, *'first chakra orientated'*. They may have been famous or infamous for their qualities of dominance, power, conquest, ambition or a driving force to express vitality and prove their virility. Rameses the Great, Pharaoh of Egypt, Builder of Egypt, father of 144 children and builder of statues and temples of Egypt, appeared to view all life from a physical perspective.

Once a psychotherapist understands the chakras, a useful tool is to understand from which chakra their clients are living their lives out of. It obviously is not healthy to be living out of only one chakra. When adults have been sexually abused as children their energy field remains small and narrow, with very little light. Adults to the victim appear large and overwhelming. Often the adult remains in the frightened energy field of the abused child, at the age they were abused. It is a task of the therapist to help the client claim back their energy field in order to prevent further abuse taking place as an adult. The client needs help, not only with the psychological problems, but with enlarging and developing their energy field to become protected.

The Second Chakra

The second chakra is orange in colour, is the emotional body where all feelings are processed. It is located over the intestines as well as part of the body's immune system. It can be a place of great distress, often where depression, seen sometimes as frozen anger, which has not been helped to melt. We need to know how we feel or don't feel about ourselves. This is the area where men and women experience many health problems. The personality of this chakra is about seven years of age, getting along with each other, sharing well and wanting others to feel as they do! It is in this chakra that we take in the feelings of others. For example, if you walk into a room where someone is very depressed you can take in the feeling of depression into this chakra and literally wonder what has hit you. It explains why we sometimes feel more exhausted with some clients more than others.

The Third Chakra

The third chakra is yellow and is the mental body or intellect. It has the personality of the twelve year old. Located over the stomach and below the sternum, it is here that thoughts, opinions and judgements are controlled. Organs here are the spleen, stomach, pancreas, liver, gall bladder, adrenals and kidneys. They control digestion—similarly these organs can be called upon to digest data that comes to them. Often the incoming data cannot be assimilated or absorbed and can lead to stomach problems and ulcers. Children assimilating so much at school often have *'tummy aches'* probably caused by the amount of information coming to them from teachers. Students taking exams often feel sick and can't digest or absorb all the information required for exam questions. It is also a place where people *'think'* about their feelings.

The Fourth Chakra

Symbolically this fourth, green chakra represents transformation of energy from the lower three chakras to a more compassionate place within ourselves. The chakra is located in the centre of the chest and is about eighteen years of age in development. This is an age where we begin to consider others before ourselves.

Although called the heart chakra, the organ most associated with it is the thymus. Conflict can internalise physical and emotional problems in this area. It may also be an area of great freedom when some of the *'rubbish'* of the lower three chakras is cleared.

The Fifth Chakra

The fifth, blue chakra is located over the throat. If difficulty of expressing oneself is experienced, it is this chakra that is affected and often causes throat problems. The age associated with this chakra is between twenty eight and thirty five. It is associated with the thyroid, which controls growth and metabolism in the human body and is controlled by speech and expression.

The Sixth Chakra

The sixth, indigo or violet chakra situated in the centre of the forehead, is often termed *the third eye*. Being on par with the brain or nervous system, it appears to be the centre of insight, intuition, awareness, sensitivity and perception. The age of this chakra personality is somewhere between forty-five and fifty. It helps to clear many problems and gives clarity on how to improve one's life. It helps each person to find more meaningful ways of living their lives, and clears blocks that may have hampered them through major life difficulties.

This chakra is the body which holds our individual future and is also our access to understanding that future. It is the realm of light, influencing all that light enables us to see. It allows us to see the light.

The Seventh Chakra

The white, seventh chakra is the ketheric body, (Kether in Hebrew simply means *'crown'*) and is located above the head. It influences the areas of consciousness known as spirit. It is the place of emergence with God, or Oneness or All. Perhaps some of the medieval painters saw auras and painted the halo above the heads of saints! But we all have a halo—maybe some are rustier than others but they are there, too!

The Prime Directive

When applying the symbology of the chakras with their personalities, lessons and distortions as taught by Rosalyn Bruyere, a different way of thinking applies to psychotherapy in which the body, mind, emotions and spirit are seen as whole person healing. The changes of consciousness and awareness in each of the chakras is vital to understanding how our bodies, emotions, mind and spirit inter-relate.

We have talked about each chakra having a personality which can assist us in finding solutions to whatever problems we have but the chakras also have a particular attitude towards reality—like the *Prime Directive* in Star Trek! Each has a purpose, a mind of its own and its going somewhere:

The First Chakra	Just is
The Second Chakra	Just feels
The Third Chakra	Just thinks and has opinions
The Fourth Chakra	Is a compassionate being
The Fifth Chakra	Just responds
The Sixth Chakra	Has insights
The Seventh Chakra	Releases and lets go

Understanding this system helps therapist and client to understand the process that is taking place, at whatever level. As this is only an introduction to the use of the chakras in psychotherapy I leave the reader to access the understanding. In 2005 Daniel Perret discussed a psychoenergetic approach to psychotherapy. He writes:

"One thing energy teaches us is that everything is connected. No energy field, no human being lives cut off or sheltered from outside influences. Studying energy brings an integrated understanding of the inside and the outside, the above and the below, spirit and matter. It teaches us how different body parts link to specific emotions, feelings, memories, thought patterns and belief structures. You do not need to see energy fields in order to work with them. We all link in to some aspects of energy. The deeper we work with someone, the more we need to be in contact with our feelings and our intuition, the more we invariably tune into non physical dimensions. We may never call it energy and that does not matter".

Conclusion

We may all be walking rainbows and not know it! The concept goes deeply into the human psyche, literally—as the biblical idea of the rainbow leaves us in awe of ancient understanding.

The colours of our own energy field are produced by our physical, emotional and mental well being alongside our heart felt feelings, self expression, perception, intuition, insight and spirituality. They govern the music we listen to, the music we compose, the colours of the clothes we wear, the environment, the need for a country walk or holiday. The pot of gold at the end of the rainbow may stand metaphorically for many other aspects of human life.

I believe the inclusion of such a wonderful system is only adding to the richness of humanity. A new definition of vocabulary and understanding creates a new agenda in the future of psychotherapy. This is already happening in the marriage of Eastern and Western cultures adding a wealth of richness to our world, not only for us now, but for the future of our children's children.

Chapter 16

GLOBAL FRACTAL WAVES

A REFLECTION

Global Fractal Waves

The most beautiful and most profound emotion we can experience is the sensation of the mystical. He to whom this emotion is a stranger, who can no longer wonder and stand rapt in awe, is as good as dead. ~Albert Einstein

Humanity has reached a stage in its evolution where the real work now has to begin. There is chaos in the world, to many, seemingly destructive, but if individuals are prepared to shift their energies, thoughts, opinions for the good of the whole, this whole new form of energy and thinking can lead to a new understanding of creative, complementary possibilities. With recent world events, organisational happenings and individual conflicts, the Editorial Board of *Inside Out* have invited me to write down my thoughts on these events, and present a constructive viewpoint of our lives and world as they are at this moment in time. There always needs to be hope in the midst of conflict and the challenge to accept tasks that are seemingly impossible!

Space Travel & The Effects Upon Mankind

Who would believe it is over forty years since man landed on the moon; the first moon landing took place on 20th July 1969. In the 1960's this was one of the greatest challenges ever to face mankind. Commander Neil Armstrong was the first man to walk on the moon and he spoke the historic words:-

'That's one small step for man, one giant leap for mankind'.

No-one knew the significance of that singular event, and the words that he spoke, and even now we are only just touching the tip of the iceberg. When men stood on the moon and looked back at planet earth they saw our home as it had never been seen before, blue and beautiful, and home. That isolated event from forty years ago has changed the way we look at our home, and advanced space technology holds great promise for the future of mankind. There has been a vast utilisation of the scientific ideas that went into space travel, now being used for the betterment of human life. Materials developed for space travel are now used in heart surgery, for heart valves; gastro problems are now being diagnosed by a Space Age capsule—the days of inserting pipes for gastro problems are over.

Ultrasound was developed in 1957, and ultrasound images taken on the space station are beamed down to earth via satellite links. Doctors on earth can diagnose any illness of the individuals on the space station. This technology is now used on earth to diagnose sports injuries and is hoped to be used by doctors in London to diagnose illnesses in isolated people in remote villages in rain forests and deserts around the world. All because humanity landed on the moon!

NASA (The National Aeronautics and Space Administration) satellite instruments, a by-product of space travel can now measure total ozone layers and ozone depleting substances. The ozone layer protects all life forms from the sun's harmful radiation. Ozone is a gas that occurs naturally in our atmosphere several miles above the surface of the earth. The Hubble telescope and the space station, alongside human ingenuity have given us a new consciousness of the earth, that it is a living, breathing organism and like human beings is healthy in areas and diseased in others.

Each one of us is earth in miniature; in fact each one of us is a universe in miniature. We are living in space, human beings, interconnected with each other, the planet and the universe in ways our consciousness would never have comprehended years ago. What happens to one of us affects another, what actions mankind make on our earth home, affects the planet. As a friend shared with me last week, she felt the planet was angry with us and was reacting energetically to humanity. For some reason the influx of complementary medicines and energy healing that have snowballed throughout Ireland in the last thirty years are here not just for making a quick buck, but with much deeper intentions which may explain the planet's condition.

Interconnectedness

However isolated individual events may seem, they are always part of a bigger plan. Underlying the isolated world of ordinary objects and human experiences are other realities. There is an interconnected world of patterns, rhythms, intertwined relationships, layer upon layer of concepts which form interconnectedness. The fact is that everything does interact with everything else, and how much of an interaction is only a matter of degree. The perception of interconnectedness of us all during spiritual practice gives flexibility to the boundaries of our own reality and helps us find our place of harmony in our world and beyond. Both modern physics and ancient Buddhist doctrine suggest that 'deep' interconnectedness embraces everything, unbound by the usual limitation of time and space.

This is where I see the great importance of the complementary medicines that now are part of everyday life in Ireland. Many of these practices are a compilation of many ancient spiritual points of view, relating to belief, cultural practices, rituals and truths originating in deeply spiritual cultures in the Near, Middle or Far East. They have given us a more profound understanding of earth energies.

The chakras which form the human energy field of the body have given us a new form of the meaning of consciousness, with the understanding that the mind is in the energy field around and through the body, which may or may not be controlled by the brain. Fantastic stuff if you make time to be with the energy of all these possibilities! Understanding the effects of radiation poisoning, disease, health and the inter-relationship of people and nations through the electronic world wide web are all part of the energy interconnectedness leading us to even greater discoveries.

The Planet As A Living Organism

This moves us into the fields of Quantum Physics, Quantum Biophysics and places energy healing to become the new medicine for the future—where energy interacts. Personal energy is connected with everything else—and each atom has its own vibrational energy. The material reality of the universe is formed by the invisible. The mind is the invisible force and in the energy fields it is the invisible moving forces that influence the physical world. Bruce Lipton in 2010 stated that the things that you cannot see shape your world and we are totally inter-related not by nature and nurture any more, but by our environment. The paradigms that we have spoken about for the last thirty or so years have happened and are continuing to happen in front of our eyes.

If, since 1969, we have seen the planet in a new light before we totally destroy it, that single act of landing on the moon may help us save our planet before our ignorance leaves our childrens' children a dying planet. We are intrinsically linked by our own very breathing of the earth's atmosphere—and the earth with ours. Is it any wonder that sickness and disease prevails both in individuals and the planet itself?

The Work Of Jean Houston

Jean Houston has influenced the development of pre- and perinatal psychology and psychotherapy through her inspirational words and work. I have taken much delight in encouraging our students to study with her.

Jean has a great gift of enabling individuals to widen their levels of consciousness in order to reach the required depth for life and also for the spiritual search for the mystic in us.

In the year 2000 I spent three weeks with Jean and her assistant Peg Rubin on her *Quest for the Grail* in England, Scotland and Wales. Her vision embracing many disciplines, guided us on a never to be forgotten journey and showed England, my place of birth, in a light that I have never see it before. A new consciousness of bringing the past and the present together for new ways of moving forward. Just as understanding our sacred journey from conception to birth can give us a new consciousness of bringing the past and the present together and helping us to move forward without unnecessary baggage.

We are being guided to the realisation that we are coming to the end of an era and beginning a new earth story. We are moving towards global civilisation and that there would be a reinvention of what human beings can be. Pre and perinatal psychotherapy has its place for new social convention; all requiring a new consciousness gestation that may never have been experienced by mankind and our planet earth

The Fractal Dimension Of Our Lives

One of Jean's greatest gifts to me in 1991 was the introduction to Fractals. I soon realised that Fractals are repetitions of the same general patterns, even the same details, at both ascending and descending scales and all that it contains is made up of folded realities within self-similar worlds. They have characteristics of self-similarity and chaos.

It appears that new technology may have discovered one of the greatest mysteries of our universe—or given us a word to describe the phenomenon of rhythms and patterns. If magnified a billion times or more it would eventually cover the universe and is really infinity. It could have been discovered anytime in history by adding and multiplying forever with very complex numbers but technology discovered it. Fractal patterns are all around us, above us and within us. Trees are fractals, with their repeated patterns of large and small branches with similar details found even in the smallest twigs. Even a single leaf shows fractal repetitions of the whole tree in both its shape and branching in its vein. In a broccoli or cauliflower you will find Fractal Geometry at its best with florets arranged in self-similarity scales. For a total fractal experience peel the leaves of an artichoke!

Fractals show a holistic hidden order behind things, which I wrote about earlier, they show a harmony in which everything affects everything else, and above all, an endless variety of interwoven patterns. In the human body these endless patterns are repeated in systems of the body, the circulatory system, the nervous system and all organs of the body.

These patterns are mirrored in the universe, from a single atom, or single cell of the human body. A spiral nebula in space that measures hundreds of light years across looks remarkably similar to something that measures a thousandth of a centimetre in the eye of a firefly! This can be seen as the fractal resonance of the other—the resonance of the microcosm of the macrocosm. It is more than probable that the chakras or human energy field of each human being mirrors the energy fields of the planet earth and that of the universe.

In 1992 I put the whole concept of fractals onto the events of a human life in my teaching of psychotherapy, discovering that there was another order of fractals present of themes that recur in the leafing and branches of happenings, events, moods, tragedies and comedies.

In my speciality of pre- and perinatal psychotherapy, putting the concept of fractals upon preconception and conception meant that our life becomes a rhythm and pattern of the state of our parents, and their lives, before our conception. And our life bears the energy or non-energy of our conception. This concept of fractals can be put on womb trauma, birth trauma, present life fractals, ancestral fractals, future life fractals and for those who believe in reincarnation, life times may recall fractal patterns depending on cause and effect. Hopefully these ideas and concepts will stretch your minds and inspire readers to think more deeply about the interconnectedness of not only planetary and global incidents but also personal and organisational happenings.

Tsunami - Natural Disasters Or Caused By Humanity?

If nature and nurture no longer have reason to be believed, environment is now seen as the controlling factor for the fate of cells, whether those of humanity and animals, or the very cells of the earth and planet. In toxic environments cells die. Put them in a healthy environment and the cells will heal themselves. Modern physics is proving that we are not victims of our own genes but a victim of our environment. It was Albert Einstein who said:-

'You cannot solve a problem with the same consciousness as the consciousness that caused the event'

These words of Einstein can be taken at any fractal level we wish to take them, and as psychotherapists listening to people's life stories daily we know how true this statement is, but how much do we take it to heart in our own lives? I'm sure in our work we may encourage clients to change the energy; that problems cannot be solved if clients are going back into the same energy in which their problems are caused. It is our own energy that needs to change in order to shift other people.

Relating previous thoughts to the latest tsunami in Japan, maybe we can all ponder on the reasons for a tsunami. The rapid displacement of the body of water takes place due to volcanic eruptions, earthquakes, underwater explosions, large meteorite impacts, mass movements above or under water and nuclear weapons testing in seas (are we really so stupid as a human race to test nuclear weapons under the seas?) Again, whether it be a natural disaster or manmade, we all know the death and destruction that is caused by a tsunami. At least ten thousand people died in the Japanese tsunami, the island has moved 2.4 metres and the planet has again shifted on its axis. This is another real wake-up call.

It was with amazement and disbelief I received the following email letter from Japan from a friend of a friend of a friend. If we are able to trace the name of the writer we will tell you but the Editorial Board decided to publish in order for these words to be read by more people. It is beautiful in its simplicity, humility and amazing culture of kindness in the face of such tragedy and devastation. As I wrote this, another earthquake measuring 7.1 hit the same area of Japan.

Letter From Japan

"Hello My Lovely Family and Friends,

First I want to thank you for your concern for me. I am very touched. I also wish to apologize for a generic message to you all. But it seems the best way at the moment to get my message to you.

Things here in Sendai have been rather surreal. But I am very blessed to have wonderful friends who are helping me a lot. Since my shack is even more worthy of that name, I am now staying at a friend's home. We share supplies like water, food and a kerosene heater. We sleep lined up in one room, eat by candlelight, and share stories. It is warm, friendly and beautiful. During the day we help each other clean up the mess in our homes. People sit in their cars, looking at news on their navigation screens, or line up to get drinking water when a source is open. If someone has water running in their homes, they put out signs so people can come to fill up their jugs and buckets.

Utterly amazingly where I am there has been no looting, no pushing in lines. People leave their front door open, as it is safer when an earthquake strikes. People keep saying, 'Oh, this is how it used to be in the old days when everyone helped one another'.

Quakes keep coming. Last night they struck about every 15 minutes. Sirens are constant and helicopters pass overhead often. We got water for a few hours in our homes last night, and now it is for half a day. Electricity came on this afternoon. Gas has yet to come on. But all of this is by area. Some people have these things, others do not. No-one has washed for several days. We feel grubby, but there are so much more important concerns that for us now. I love this peeling away of non-essentials. Living fully on the level of instinct, of intuition, of caring, of what is needed for survival, not just of me, but of the entire group.

There are strange parallel universes happening. Houses are a mess in some places, yet then a house with futons or laundry drying out in the sun. People lining up for water and food, and yet a few people out walking their dogs. All happening at the same time. Other unexpected touches of beauty are first, the silence at night. No cars. No-one out on the streets. And the heavens at night are scattered with stars. I usually can only see about two, but now the whole sky is filled. The mountains of Sendai are solid and with the crisp air we can see them silhouetted against the sky magnificently.

And the Japanese themselves are so wonderful. I come back to my shack to check on it each day, now to send this email since the electricity is on, and I find food and water left in my entranceway. I have no idea from whom, but it is there. Old men in green hats go from door to door checking to see if everyone is OK. People talk to complete strangers asking if help is needed. I see no sign of fear. Resignation, yes, but fear or panic, no.

They tell us we can expect aftershocks, and even other major quakes, for another month or more. And we are getting constant tremors, rolls, shaking, rumbling. I am blessed that I live in a part of Sendai that is a bit elevated, a bit more solid than other parts. So, so far this area is better off than other. Last night my friend's husband came in from the country bringing food and water. Blessed again.

Somehow at this time I realise from direct experience that there is indeed an enormous cosmic evolutionary step that is occurring all over the world right at this moment. And somehow as I experience the events happening now in Japan, I can feel my heart opening very wide. My brother asked me if I felt so small because all this is happening. I don't. Rather I feel as part of something happening that is much larger than me. This wave of birthing (worldwide) is hard and yet magnificent.

Thank you again for your care and love of me, With love, in return..."

The Microcosm Of The Macrocosm

It was Bruce Lipton, on a visit to Dublin who said:-

"You are the creator of your life and you can create what you want when you get the new knowledge. When you become conscious you become the driver—if you are not conscious or aware you are less connected to the field. Negative thoughts will create negative experiences. Positive thoughts will harmonise and create positive actions. You bring into your life what you are focusing on."

The isolated events that happen in our lives cause other events to happen on fractal levels that seriously affect the lives of others.

Worldwide Uncertainty

Worldwide, societies are crying out for assistance in the transformation of people, organisations, institutions and governments. As Jean Houston describes it so aptly, when she comments that too many problems in societies stem today, in part, from leadership that is ill-prepared to deal with present complexities. This is not just a matter of inadequate training in the realities of global change, but even more tragically, a lack of human resourcefulness; leaders living out of a field of awareness that is both limited and limiting in their abilities to deal with the world as it is today.

The human race needs leaders and strong people, conceived and born consciously who can rise to any challenge effectively. Those to be parents willing to listen to events and experiences from the womb, will birth new lives who will be able to rise to the challenges of our new millennium. It is known that leaders, like most of society, emerge as highly compromised versions of what we could be. The state of the world reflects this in a most dangerous way. The absence in the world of skilled facilitators and leaders is alarming—otherwise there would not be such chaos in countries, governments and organisations. We have new knowledge and new technologies, of which conscious parenting, conscious conception and awareness of life in the womb is vital. Skilled leaders with the courage to lead the shift to new values and practices with the strength of their conviction, are needed to stop the carnage as Frank Lake warned of 40 years ago.

Reflections For The Future

Leadership today, on any fractal, is caught uncertain and unprepared with too much happening too quickly. We need CPD trainings to help us prepare for the new world, led by those who know what they are talking about. The re-patterning of human nature and the re-genesis of society are forces that push us to use more than 10% of our brain to make us possible humans. Psychotherapists attend creative workshops, or run them, but the larger picture of why we attend workshops is not just to get hours for accreditation, but to expand our energy fields to find that interconnectedness in ourselves, families, organisations, nations and the world. We have studied the collective unconscious and behaviour patterns, experienced meditation and visualisation, know our psychological histories, listen daily to people's stories and are capable of empathising with our fellow humans. We are capable of understanding interconnectedness, but not until this is realised will we take that step into the future, confident of great possibilities.

My reflection has led me into energy fields deep in my subconscious that I hope will be helpful in your life. Given the opportunities and trainings that may become available we can learn to think, feel and know in new ways. With more awareness we may become more creative, more imaginative and reach realistic limits that help us all deal with the complex challenges of life.

On that fractal level, everything we do and learn is not there solely for our own purpose, but for the good of the whole, as in the examples I have given. No event stands alone and the fractal waves of our lives and others are interconnected.

We are a constantly learning society but we have to rise above our humanity and bring in the divine, whatever that might be for us. Our own sacredness for living in these tumultuous times is a must to get us through. The future lies in our hands, individuals completing the gestalt with more thought for wholeness and less of the super ego, selfishness and narcissism. At whatever fractal level, we need to get out of the crisis programme and pull our energy out of old-world thinking and systems that are not working. The usual formulas and stopgap solutions born in an earlier era will not help, nor heal us. What a task, what a challenge! This is where the real work is to be done.

Chapter 17

THE WAY FORWARD

The Way Forward

As we come to the end of our journey through pre- and perinatal psychotherapy, we become conscious of how far we have come and how far we have yet to go. It seems fitting to take a broader perspective on the issues of life before birth as they are reflected in human life everywhere. Human life can become a dangerous structure if it is driven by negative fractals from the womb. Clearly, if we remove or change these fractals, we can make a fundamental positive difference to the lives of people everywhere.

The Holistic Therapies

Our expanded consciousness, and a more holistic view of the world that we discussed in the previous chapter, has been accompanied by the development of a new, more holistic style of psychology. Psychology is understood to be the study of the psyche, mind, consciousness or soul. It has needed to become scientific over the years in order to measure, to validate and to objectify. It tended to turn away from the intangibles of human experiences like emotions, feelings and aesthetic values concentrating on more specific aspects of behaviour. As in all things psychology is at its peak of ebbing and flowing! Personality psychology is on the move, in keeping with modern day humanity.

Social changes and human behaviour now point to a distinct shift. Connell says this awareness is now leading to:

A psychology that emphasises growth, not adjustment; the unique, not the normal; and the creative, not the average.

This branch of evolving psychology is called Humanistic Psychology, Third Force Psychology or Existential Psychology. It emphasises the breathing, living, loving, sensing, multi-faceted human being. This human person is more than a statistic; more than a laboratory rat; more than a name and number in a research filing system.

The Association of Humanistic Psychologists (AHP)

Carl Rogers said in the early 1960s:

"If the human species is to survive at all on this globe, the human being must become more readily adaptive to new problems and situations; must be able to select that which is valuable for development and survival out of new and complex situations, must be accurate in his appreciation of reality if he is to make such selections."

Along with Abraham Maslow, Rollo May and others Rogers went on to form the AHP in 1962 in USA. It leads the way in the development and dissemination of information to expand personal and social consciousness. Being the *'third force'* in psychology, Humanistic Psychology is not seen as a specific style of therapy but more a philosophy, in which many specific modalities share a common set of values, which are to promote personal growth, human potential, self-determination and self-actualisation.

Today, in our Global village, we are engrossed in our own development, with a greater understanding of the expansion of the human mind. We are reaching out to acquire a better way of life for all people. Humanistic Psychology is seen as an excellent way of approaching this evolution. It has emerged as a result of dissatisfaction with the rigid, Freudian psychoanalytical and behaviourist approach to people. It takes a more optimistic view, regarding human beings as fundamentally good and as having huge potential, which is distorted when personal and social needs are not met.

Creative People

The value of our differences, cultures, behaviour, religion, dress, life styles, opinions and much more is now acceptable. Creativity is encouraged, and research on creative human beings has been ongoing. Results show that they have an ability to integrate the higher functions of love and service to others. They are more able to think and act autonomously and this behaviour is known as *self-actualisation*. The person who achieves self-actualisation in a constructive and significant way, is a great asset to humanity. Those who use their creativity in a destructive and aggressive way are not—they are picked out by the media to show how bad it is to become involved in such things.

Highly creative people are not selfish, in that they seek only their own growth. But they wish to develop the growth of others who share and participate in their lives. Personal freedom does not mean having a license to do whatever they wish. The distinction between liberty and license is crucial. License lacks the essential ingredients of responsibility, whereas liberty assumes self-governance. Humanistic psychology enables a person to grow and heal through his or her own individual process.

A Set Of Principles Of Humanistic Psychology

The AHP states that the centrally held views of humanistic and holistic principles of psychology are:

1. It is necessary to emphasise the importance of the whole person; wholeness or holiness as described by some, reached by integrating five levels of consciousness—namely body, mind, feelings/emotions, behaviour and spirit.
2. That psychology is a total overview of human experience.
3. Experience and its meaning are the primary realities in human psychology, and that experience is essential for the understanding of all people.
4. All people are basically creative.
5. Psychology affirms the importance and uniqueness of human life.
6. Choice, self-realisation, spontaneity, love, creativity, valuing, responsibility, authenticity, meaning, transcendental experience and courage are valid for psychological study but unacceptable in most other systems.
7. Psychology includes social change and concern for the way in which individuals are helped or hindered in their growth.

Integration

Many people now working in the field of Humanistic Psychology are unaware that they are doing anything that is different. Young people are joining self-development groups because they are a recognised part of their society. Businesses and industry send their directors, members, workers and staff on Humanistic Psychology conferences and workshops to improve them not only as people, but to encourage a finer quality of task force and business.

Those now working in the field as therapists, counsellors, healers, those who teach and practise alternative therapies and medicines, do so by having experienced their own difficulties in life, perhaps physical illness, disease and stressful traumas. Their health and well being, they have taken on as their personal responsibility—the traditional dependency upon orthodox medicine and the doctor is no longer uppermost in their minds. A major advantage of so many more available types of treatment means the finer points of different alternative therapies may be integrated with the finest in technological medicine, in order to achieve healing instead of the model of utilising only one school of thought.

One usually finds out about this integration through individual work and experience, and not purely by intellect and theory, although each does have its place. Often there is not a set system or any formal training to follow. The experience in groups is often the only direction.

Medical vs Humanistic Models

There are fundamental differences between the medical and humanistic models of sickness, in the body/mind—or both are one in the holistic model. One focuses on sickness and health, the other on education—growth. One believes that the patient is ill and needs to be cured, while the other believes that people seek out a chance for personal growth and development.

In the medical model, drugs are prescribed. In the other, complementary therapies and medicines are sought. The one describes disease, symptoms and diagnosis. The other talks about experiential learning, self-actualisation and human potential.

We can have a problem-orientated approach or an exploratory approach. Illness can be something to get well from, or something to journey through, towards wholeness and integration.

The healthy doctor treats the sick patient, but the humanistic therapist and client are both equal human beings. In the medical field the traditional authority of doctor is paramount, while the humanistic therapeutic relationship is more equal.

A doctor assumes an anonymous, detached safe and protected stance, but the humanistic therapist is necessarily more real and authentic, vulnerable and exposed. Traditional therapy is limited to talking and verbal communication but in experiential therapy there is learning and emotions expressed.

Holistic Health

The Holistic Health paradigm began to emerge in the early 1970's as part of a non-drug response to the psychedelic exploration undertaken in the 1960's. Alternative health care is now available, not as a threat or in opposition to orthodox medical methods but to work hand in hand to provide a holistic approach to people.

Although Humanistic Psychology originally started as a 'third force' in relation to psychoanalysis and behaviourism and did not adopt the model—it does not have to be rejected. The two models may be integrated without threat to either side.

It is often insecurity and fear or fear of insecurity that causes some people to heavily criticise *the other side* without researching the necessary facts. Complementary and preventative medicines, alternative therapies and orthodox medicine can work side by side for the integrative healing of body, mind and spirit. But it is understandably difficult to expose oneself to other methods when trained and entrenched in a particular school of therapy. The flexibility and adaptability that Carl Rogers spoke of in the 1960's is never more needed than now.

There is now a Growth Movement, where individuals engage in a wide variety of activities concerned with personal growth—or realising the full potential of the individual to improve the quality of life in society as a whole. Humanistic Psychology, and primal integration, are part of that movement.

Awakening Spirituality

The essential message emerging from Jean Houston and other great thinkers of this century is that not only can we find the human potential within us, but also the sacredness and spirituality which are often latent within our being.

The spiritual awakening in our present time must be differentiated from a *'religious revival'*. It has not grown out of the church or conventional western religions. It is eclectic, drawing from a wide range of eastern and western systems, and focused on the expansion of human consciousness.

The Christian churches particularly have traditionally been suspicious of anything that suggests a connection with non-Christian eastern religions, lumping them together with the occult, esoteric and paganism. Perhaps it might be reasoned here that ignorance is the only sin. It is important also to realise that a certain proportion of the population have jumped on the New Age fantasy bandwagon and have avoided the reality that life actually does also have its difficulties. The gestalt needs to be completed in order that we are not left unbalanced.

A Therapeutic Path For Mankind

I believe that the Humanistic and Integrative therapeutic path is of enormous value for the future of mankind. John Rowan explains that we reach a more enlightened spiritual deepening within ourselves by experiencing various types of therapies evolving today. The spiritual is reached by knowing ourselves. Again this is suspect when individuals go immediately into meditation, spiritual practices and becoming *'holy'* or *'pious'* without having looked at the darker side. This approach puts over a false, dishonest and somewhat suspicious aura that questions its authenticity. This is what I believe the critics find objectionable.

The therapeutic path that our clients walk with us based in the study of uterine life and the experience of birth and how these stages of development affect our emotional, social and psychological wellbeing. The pre- and Perinatal Psychology Association of North America was founded by Thomas Verny MD and David Chamberlain PhD, in the early 1980s. This organisation (now APPPAH, The Association for Prenatal and Perinatal Psychology and Health) is dedicated to the in-depth exploration of the psychological dimension of human reproduction and pregnancy and the mental and emotional development of the unborn and newborn child. It is a holistic, multi-disciplinary association of people from diverse backgrounds such as obstetrics, midwifery, nursing, perinatology, paediatrics, childbirth education, psychology, psychiatry, law, the clergy, ethology, anthropology, counselling, teaching, therapy, and concerned parents.

The common denominator amongst this diverse group is the belief that the way in which we were conceived, the process of growing in our mothers' wombs are all part of our unconscious affective memory, and influences our life long behaviour.

A Pioneer

As a Pre- and Perinatal Psychotherapist and healer, I have struggled to pioneer such a belief, when the majority of the human race in this century, have worked on the assumption that babies begin to live, breathe, pay attention, see, hear sense and play only after birth.

The belief is that the first five years of life are the most important. When Dr. Thomas Verny wrote his challenging book, *The Secret Life of the Unborn Child* he took a remarkable and controversial look at life before birth. The result of twenty years of painstaking research into the earliest stages of life, this testimony and Dr. Verny's evidence of intelligent life in the womb is overwhelming.

Whatever our beliefs in this field, there is a hard core of knowledge emerging in which David Chamberlain has led the field with his extraordinary discoveries in scientific and medical research. He has presented scientific evidence showing that even in the womb the foetus experiences a wide variety of emotions, that the seemingly random noises new-borns make, are conscious attempts to communicate; and that cognition and reasoning are more highly developed than we have previously believed.

Empirical evidence of consciousness in the prenate is available, in order that we might fully accept subjective accounts. This empirical evidence for birth and prenatal activity, consciousness and memory, comes from an abundance of sources documented in 1991 by Michael Irving, who is working energetically to accumulate many sources world-wide to provide researchers with as much evidence as they require.

We have reached the point that the evidence has become controvertible, however hard it may be to believe. At the moment we have only the incredulity of some people, who think they know better, standing between us and the chance to make a substantive difference to human suffering. We have developed excellent methods to heal prenatal trauma, which is accessible and which works well. As a corollary to this, for more than seventy years, alongside the development of these therapies, has been the idea of prevention of birth trauma by changing the way that babies are conceived, carried and delivered.

The End Of An Era

The lecture Jean Houston delivered, entitled *Preparing the Foetus, Repairing the Earth,* which gave me the idea of transposing fractals in pre- and perinatal work, can change the nature of prebirth fractals forever. Her vision, embracing so many disciplines, is guiding us to the realisation that we are coming to the end of an era. She reminds us that we are coming to the beginning of a new earth story: we are moving towards global civilisation. She emphasised strongly that here is a chance to reinvent what humans can be: here is a critical meaning or new social convention, requiring a new conscious gestation that has never taken place before in this way in the history of mankind and our planet Earth.

People in the Pre- and Perinatal field are proving, in whatever role they participate, that:

How we are prepared for conception; the circumstances surrounding our conception; the state of our parents at our conception; how we are treated in the womb; how we are born—influences our lifelong behaviour, and that conclusively, we live our lives according to the trauma or glory or our birth.

This is the consciousness concerning childbirth that needs to be infiltrated not slowly, but gently, into the human psyche. We are born one way or another, and this dictates our life imprints. If we are to understand our human nature and care for our planet, we must understand our beginnings and believe and know that each individual has a personal responsibility for the fate of our home, Earth.

The way we live our lives affects the way in which we treat our planet. No one can look after our planet but us. The pregnant world situation is not unlike a vast womb of gestation. Everything is in a foetal state of preparation before regenesis. All the old systems are breaking down—because before you go into transition everything has to break down.

What Can We Do?

We are born from dust and return to dust. We are living and spiritual beings belonging to the Earth. To understand the way in which we were conceived, and conceive, is of the utmost importance, covering vast topics of human understanding. Earth is hurting and no one but us is responsible. For mother Earth to avoid the greatest miscarriage of all time, or to deliver the greatest gift to future generations, is in our hands.

Children conceived in love, are loving; in fear, are fearful; in hate, know only hate; in violence, become violent; in peace, are peaceful. We have so much to learn from each other across all disciplines of conceiving, bearing, birthing and rearing the children of the future.

May we teach each other how to deliver peace and be open to every area where we can work in harmony.

Conception To Birth

Take seriously the research that is rapidly growing from hundreds of researchers in diverse aspects of pre- and Perinatal Psychology throughout the world. In our experiential psychotherapy we discover, in the depths of the human psyche, aspects of human nature that are much deeper, and go further back than is comfortable for many people to perhaps want to know. As human race, we have much to learn, and more to take responsibility for. It is said that ignorance is the only sin. Parents, psychologists, the medical profession, all of us have treated the earliest period of human development—from preconception to birth—as an insensitive, unconscious, unfeeling period of growth. Babies are teaching us the opposite.

We need to realise that the time in the womb is crucial and that the painful and life-threatening experiences associated with pregnancy abuse and the passage through the birth canal naturally provoke a corresponding violent response. They act as a psychic draw to later life situations. Teach mothers-to-be that emotions of deep anger can be dissipated in the womb.

If mother is aware of her own emotions and owns them, the foetus does not have to imbibe them. Even though the foetus may feel the anger, the clarity of who the anger belongs to, can lessen the impact on the foetus. The love of the mother and father can help to decrease the impact of outside anger and tensions. This good, understanding parenting is essential. No parent really wants their child to suffer.

Discuss seriously whether changed birthing and childcaring methods would prevent violent acts of crimes and war. Leboyer was a major force in the argument towards more gentle birthing methods. He taught that violent births breed violence, gentleness breeds gentleness and peace encourages peace.

This Early Research Is FACT

Newborn babies and also adults who were traumatised in this early period are teaching us. These early imprinting memories arise when the problems presented by people are related to these areas. This repository of aggressive, angry tendencies is harboured in the unconscious for the rest of our lives, until or unless we make an effort to confront them of transform them in some variety of self exploration. From the field of experiential psychotherapy the answer to the cycles of violence, war and death-rebirth is to stop the acting out, and relive these cycles of violence at their preconception, conception and pre and perinatal origins—in order to find peace.

War And Violence

Although not all anger comes from the pre- and perinatal time, work in our field of pre- and Perinatal Psychotherapy over the years throws an entirely new light on the forms of human violence perpetrating the global crisis. Violence is displayed in the form of wars, riots, murder, torture, terrorism and crime, all of which seem to be escalating. Many of these forms of violence can only come from individuals collectively. War would be the greatest struggle between nations.

National leaders may take us into war as they act out their own perinatal dynamics in gruesome ways—and others follow their own dynamics. These are so hidden, repressed and overlaid with defences that the conscious mind has absolutely no access to them as being part of ones unconscious. The conscious mind is completely able to convince itself that those dynamics are actual, real and doubtless part of the situation and requires an actual, real and extreme response.

Lloyd de Mause the psychohistorian says bluntly that groups, wherever, whether face to face or historical, induce a, *"foetal trance state"* in their numbers, reawakening memories from uterine and perinatal life. We would now add to this, conception.

Happier Conceptions Make A Happier World

We are coming to the beginning of a new earth story—we are moving towards global civilisation in the next millennium. A new conscious gestation is required that has never taken place before in the history of mankind and our planet.

This consciousness is necessary to understand that how we are prepared for before conception; the state of our parents when we are conceived; how we are treated in the womb and how we are born influences our life-long behaviour. Driven by fractals from the womb, we live our lives according to the trauma, or glory, of our conception and our birth.

~ The End ~

BIBLIOGRAPHY

Adzema, M.D., (1996) *The Scenery of Healing*. Commentary on De Mause's Restaging of Fetal Trauma in War and Social Violence. *pre- and Perinatal Journal* Vol 10 No 4 pp 261-272

American Psychiatric Association (1994) *Diagnostic And Statistical Manual Of Mental Disorders*, Fourth edition. Washington, DC. American Psychiatric Association.

Axline, V., (1969) *Play Therapy*, New York, Ballatine Books.

Baker, J., Parvati and Frederick, A. (1986) *Conscious Conception*. Elemental Journey through the Labyrinth of Sexuality. North Atlantic Books. USA

Barker, D., (1998) *Mothers, Babies and Health in Later Life*. Research Data from the Medical Research Centre, Southampton University. Churchill Livingstone, UK

Boklage, C.E. (1990) *Survival Probability of Human Conceptions From Fertilisation To Term*. International Journal of Fertility Vol.35 No.2

Bowlby, J.A. (2000) *A Secure Base; Parent-Child Attachment and Healthy Development*. Basic Books: New York

Breuer, J., S. Freud, (1895) *Studies on Hysteria*. Translated by James Strachey.

Breuer, J., S. Freud, (1895) *The Psychical Mechanism of Hysterical Phenomena*. Paper translated (1909)

Brown, I.G. & Somers, B.,(2002) *Journey in Depth: A Transpersonal Perspective Book*. Archive Publishing.

Bruyere, R.L., (1989) *Wheels of Light*. Ed. Jeanne Farrens. Fireside Books, Simon and Schuster, New York

Bruyere, R.L., (1990) *Chakra Healing*. Audio Renaissance Tapes LA, USA

Caldwell, C. (1999) *Dying To Be Born and Being Born to Die*: Cell Death As A Defining Pattern in Human Development. Journal of Pre and Perinatal Psychology and Health. Vol. 13

Campbell, S., (2004) *Watch Me Grow*. A unique 3-dimensional, week-by-week look at baby's behaviour and development in the womb. Carroll and Brown Ltd.

Carter, L., (2005) *Enough About You, Let's Talk About Me*. How to recognise and manage the Narcissists in your life. Jossey Bass, San Francisco.

Chamberlain, D., (1990) *The Expanding Boundaries of Memory*. Journal for pre- and Perinatal Psychology and Health. Vol 4(3)

Chamberlain, D., (1995) *Paper Observations of Behaviour Before Birth; Current Findings*. May. 11th, International Conference of ISPPM. Heidelberg.

Chamberlain, D., (1996) *Life In The Womb, Danger and Opportunities*. Journal for Pre- and Perinatal Psychology and Health. Vol 14 No 1-2 p.37

Chamberlain, D., (1998) *The Mind of Your Newborn Baby*. North Atlantic Books, Berkeley, California. (Previously published as Babies Remember Birth (1998) by Tarcher, LA, USA.)

Chamberlain, D., (1998) *The Mind of Your Newborn Baby*. North Atlantic Books. USA

Chamberlain, D., (2013) *Windows to the Womb; Revealing the Conscious Baby From Conception to Birth*. North Atlantic Books, Berkeley, California.

Christian, Carol (1991) *In The Spirit of Truth*. A Reader in the Work of Frank Lake. Darton, Longman and Todd, London.

Cole, J. (2008) *No-one Knows*. The true story of the secret survivor. Borderline Personality Disorder. Published privately. www.proofreading.com www.secretsurvivor.com

Crowe, J., (2000) *Birthing a Vision for the Future*. Network, Vol 35, County Clare, Ireland.

Davies, B.(2002) *Journey of the Soul*. Hodder and Stoughton: London

Docker-Drysdale, B., (1968) *Therapy In Child Care*, London, Longmans.

Docker-Drysdale, B., (1971) *Consultations in Childcare*, London, Longmans.

Emerson, W., (1984) *Infant And Child Birth Refacilitation*, HPR, California.

Erikson, E.H., (1950) *Childhood and Society*. Pelican Books.

Farmer, S. (1989) *Adult Children of Abusive Parents*. Ballantine: New York

Farrant, G., (1988) *Cellular Consciousness and Conception*, pre- and Perinatal News, Vol. 2, No. 2 (From PPPANA 2162 Ingleside Ave. Macon, Georgia 3120)

Feldmar, A., (1979) *The Embryology of Consciousness*. What is a normal pregnancy? The Psychological Aspects of Abortion. Eds. D.Mall and W.Watts, Washington, DC; University Publications of America.

Fodor, N., (1949) *The Search for the Beloved; A Clinical Investigation of The Trauma of Birth and Prenatal Conditioning*. University Books, New York. USA.

Fodor, N., (1969) *Analyst of the Unexplained: Allen Spraggett*. Psychoanalytic Review, Vol.54 pp.128-137

Franzek, E. J. et al. (2008) *Prenatal Exposure to the 1944-45 Dutch 'hunger winter' and addiction in later life*. Addiction No. 103

Freud, S., (1900) *Interpretation of Dreams*.

Freud, S., (1915) *Collected Papers*, Volume 111

Gabriel, M., (1992) *Voices From The Womb*. Aslan. Lower Lake, CA 95457

Gilliland, A.L., T. Verny (1999) *The Effects of Domestic Abuse on the Unborn Child*. pre- and Perinatal Psychology Journal, Vol 13 (3-4)

Ginnott, H.,(1961) *Group Psychotherapy With Children*, New York, McGraw Hill.

Grant, E., (1980) *The Effect Of Smoking On Pregnancy and Children*, in Guidelines for Future Parents, Foresight, APPCC. Surrey.

Grof, S. & C. Grof., (1990) *The Stormy Search for the Self*. Hayton,

Grof, S., (1975) *Realms of the Human Unconscious*, Viking Press.

Grof, S., (1985) *Beyond the Brain Death and Transcendence in Psychotherapy*. State University of New York Press.

Grof, S., & H.Z. Bennet. (1992) *The Holotropic Mind; The Three Levels of Human Consciousness and How They Shape Our Lives*. Harper, San Francisco.

Hayton, A., (2003, 2007) *Unpublished material*. www.wombtwin.com

Hayton, A., (2011) *Womb Twin Survivors*. Wren Publications. St Albans, UK.

Hayton, A., (Ed) (2007) *Untwinned: Perspectives on the Death of a Twin Before Birth*, Wren Publications.

Hayton, A., (Ed) (2008) *A Silent Cry: Womb Twin Survivors Tell Their Stories*. Wren Publications. St Albans, UK. Tarcher/Perigree USA.

Herman, J. L. (1992) *Trauma and Recovery*. Basic Books. Harper Collins: New York

Hoek, H.W., A. S. Brown, E. Susser, (1998) *The Dutch Famine and Schizophrenia Spectrum Disorders; Prenatal nutritional deficiencies as cause for neurodevelopmental disorders at the end of World War 2*. Society of Psychiatry Epidemiology No.33

Hotchkiss, S., (2002) *Why Is It Always About You? The Seven Deadly Sins Of Narcissism*, Free Press. Simon and Schuster, New York, USA.

Houston J., (1982) *The Possible Human*. JP Tarcher, Los Angeles.

Houston J., (1987) *The Search for the Beloved; Journeys In Sacred Psychology*. JP Tarcher, Los Angeles.

Houston, J., (1996) *A Mythic Life Learning to Live Our Greater Story*. Harper, San Francisco.

Houston, J., (2006) *Social Artistry. Discovering the Creative Dimensions of Leadership*. Jean Houston. Ashland, Oregon 97520

International and Universal Press. UK.

Irving, M.C., (1991) *Literature Review And Bibliography Of pre- and Perinatal Psychology and Art Therapy*. Carriage House Studios, Toronto. Canada.

Jackins, H. (1965) *The Human Side of Human Beings*. Rational Island: Seattle. USA

Jacobson B. and M. Bygdeman (1998) *Obstetric Care and Proneness of Offspring to Suicide as Adults: A Case Control Study*. British Medical Journal, Vol. 317 no. 7169.

James, W., (1890) *Principles of Psychology*.

Janov, A., (1973) *The Feeling Child*, Simon and Schuster.

Johnson, V., (1971) *Neonatal Experiences and Psychopathology*, Society for Neuroscience, Houston.

Judith, A., (1996) *Eastern Body, Western Mind; Psychology and the Chakra System*, Celestial Arts, USA.

Kalshed D. (1996) *The Inner World of Trauma*. Routledge: London

Kenworthy, M., (1928) *The Prenatal And Early Postnatal Phenomena of Consciousness*, in The Unconscious; A Symposium.(1966) Books for Libraries Press.

K, S.(2011). Alison Hunter in conversation with Sarah Kay. *Inside Out*, 65, 2-27. Retrieved 30 December 2018 from https://iahip.org/inside-out/issue-65-autumn-2011/alison-hunter-in-conversation-with-sarah-kay

Lake, B., (1983) *Remembering Frank.* Contact.

Lake, F., (1966) *Clinical Theology.* DLT: London

Lake, F., (1978) *Treating Psychosomatic Disorders Related to Birth Trauma.* Journal of Psychosomatic Research No. 22 pp. 227—238.

Lake, F., (1980) *Studies in Constricted Confusion—Exploration of a pre- and Perinatal Paradigm,* Oxford, CTA.

Lake, F., (1981) *Studies in Constricted Confusion; Epigrammatic Charts,* Clinical Theology Association. Nottingham, England.

Lake, F., (1981) *Tight Corners in Pastoral Counselling.* Darton, Longman and Todd (Reprinted (2005) Bridge Pastoral Foundation, Birmingham, UK.

Lake, F., (1982) *Mutual Caring.* Unpublished paper. (Edited (1998) by David Wasdell entitled, *The First Trimester* published by URCHIN) Lake, F., (1966) Clinical Theology, Darton, Longman and Todd, London, UK.

Lake, F., (1982) *With Respect; A Doctor's Response To A Healing Pope.* Darton, Longman and Todd, London.

Larsson, G., M. Eriksson, Zetterstrom (1979) *Amphetamine Addiction and Pregnancy, Psycho-social and Medical Aspects.* Dept of Pediatrics. Karolinska Institute, St Gorans Children's Hospital, Stockholm, Sweden.

Lee, E., S. Cole-Harding (2001) *The Effects of Prenatal Stress and of Alcohol and Nicotine Exposure on Human Sexual Orientation.* Physiology and Behaviour No. 74, pp. 213-226.

Levine, P. and Kline, M. (2007) *Trauma Through a Child's Eyes.* North Atlantic Books: USA

Levine, P. with Frederick, A. (1997) *Waking the Tiger.* North Atlantic Books. USA

Linnell, M., (1990) *Relating to the Chakras.* Self and Society Vol 21 No 6.

Lipton, Bruce, (2005) *The Biology of Belief; Unleashing The Power of Consciousness, Matter and Miracles.* Mountain of Love/ Elite Books, Santa Rosa, CA 95404

Lipton, Bruce, and S. Bhaerman, (2010) *Spontaneous Evolution; Our Positive Future And A Way To Get There From Here.* Hay House. UK

Lowen, A., (1985) *Narcissism; Denial of the True Self.* Touchstone, Simon and Schuster.

Lyman, BJ., (2007) *Prenatal and Birth Memories.* S.B.G.I. Santa Barbara, CA 93102-4214

Lyman, BJ., (2007) *Prenatal and Perinatal Psychotherapy with Adults: An Integrative Model for Empirical Testing.* Santa Barbara Graduate Institute: USA

Maret, S.M. (1992) *Frank Lake's Maternal-Fetal Distress Syndrome; An Analysis.* (Dissertation submitted to the Graduate School of Drew University in partial fulfilment of the requirements for the Degree of Doctor of Philosophy.)

Masterson, J.F., (1981) *The Narcissistic and Borderline Disorders; An Integrated Developmental Approach.* Routledge. New York. USA.

Masterson, J.F., (2000) *The Personality Disorders; A New Look At The Developmental Self and Object Relations Approach.* Zeig Tucker and Co. Phoenix, Arizona. USA.

Mauger, B. (2008) *Love in a Time of Broken Heart*. Soul Connections: Dublin

McAll, K.,(1982) *Healing the Family Tree*, Sheldon Press.

McBride, K., (2008) *Will I Ever be Good Enough? Healing the Daughters of Narcissistic Mothers*. Free Press. New York. USA.

McCarty, W.A., (2009) *Welcoming Consciousness*. W.B.P. Santa Barbara, CA 93109

Moss, R.S. (1983) *Frank Lake's Maternal-Foetal Distress Syndrome*. Primal Integration Workshops, Oxford, CTA.

Mott, F.J., (1965) *The Universal Design of Creation*, Mark Beech, Edenbridge, UK.

Mott, F.J., (1969) *The Nature Of The Self*, The Integration Publishing Company, London, UK.

Mott, F.J., (1970) *The Little History*, Mark Beech, Edenbridge, England.

Mott. F.J., (1952) *Play Therapy With Children*, The Integration Publishing Company, UK.

Motz, J., (1998) *Hands of Life*. Bantam Books. USA.

Napier, N. (1993) *Getting Through The Day*. Strategies for Adults Hurt as Children. Norton: New York and London

Nathanielsz, P., (1992) *Life Before Birth And A Time to be Born*. Promethean Press, Ithaca, New York.

Nathanielsz, P., (1999) *Life in the Womb: The Origin of Health and Disease*. Promethean Press, Ithaca, New York.

Nelson, J.E., (1994) *Healing The Split: Integrating Spirit Into Our Understanding Of The Mentally Ill*. University State of New York.

Noble, E., (1993) *Primal Connections: How Our Experiences From Conception To Birth Influence Our Emotions, Behaviour and Health*. Simon Schuster. Fireside Books.

O'Moore, M., (1994) *Handbook On Bullying*, Trinity College, Dublin.

Oaklander, V., (1978) *Windows to our Children: A Gestalt Therapy Approach To Children And Adolescents*. Real People Press, Moab, Utah.

Paul. A.M. (2010) *Origins: How The Nine Months Before Birth Shape The Rest Of Our Lives*. Hay House, Inc.

Peerbolte, LM, (1954) *Prenatal Dynamics*, Leiden. Sitjhoff's Uitgeversmaatschappij, N.V.

Peerbolte, LM, (1975) *Psychic Energy In Prenatal Dynamics*, Parapsychology, Peak Experiences. Severe Publishers, Wassenaar.

Penfield. W., (1976) *The Mystery of the Mind*, Princeton University Press.

Perret, D., (2005) *The Five Elements in Therapy: A Psychoenergetic Approach to Psychotherapy and Music Therapy*. Inside Out, Vol 46.

Pert, CB., (1997/2003) *Molecules of Emotion: Why You Feel the Way You Feel*. Scribner. New York.

Pert, CB., (2000) *Your Body Is Your Subconscious Mind, Your Brain Is Not In Charge*. (Audio) Sounds True, Colorado.

Pert, CB., (2003) *Molecules of Emotion: The Science Behind Mind Body Medicine*. Scribner, USA.

Peters, J., (1989) *Frank Lake, The Man and His Work*. Darton, Longman and Todd, London.

Radin, D., (1997) *The Conscious Universe*, Harper Collins.

Rank, O.,(1929) *The Trauma of Birth*. Routledge and Kegan Paul Ltd. (Originally published (1923) Publisher unknown. Reprinted (1973) Harper Torchbook edition, Harper and Row. New York. Also reprinted (1993) Dover Publications. New York.)

Reich, W., (1948) *The Discovery Of The Orgone*. Vol 1. Orgone Institute Press, USA.

Rowan, J., (1993) *Transpersonal Psychotherapy And Counselling*. Routledge.

Rowan, J., & Dryden, W.,(1988) *Integrative Therapy in Britain*.

Salk, L.,(1966) *Thoughts on the Concept of Imprinting and its Place in Early Human Development*, Canadian Psychiatric Association Journal No. 11.

Solomon, M. and Siegal, D. J. (Ed) (2003) *Healing Trauma*. Norton: New York

Tubridy, A., (2003) *When Panic Attacks*. New Leaf, Gill and Macmillan.

Tuormaa, T. E., (1994) *The Adverse Effects of Alcohol on Reproduction*. Produced by the Association For The Promotion of Pre Conceptual Care, Surrey.

Vaughan, F., (1986) *The Inward Arc*. Healing And Wholeness In Psychology And Spirituality. New Science Library, Shambala.

Verny, T. & J. Kelly, (1981) *The Secret Life of the Unborn Child*, Sphere Books Ltd. UK.

Verny. T.R. (Ed.), (1987) *Pre and Perinatal Psychology*, An Introduction. Human Sciences. New York.

Verny. T.R., (2000) *Nurturing The Unborn Child*. Olmstead Press, Chicago, IL.

Ward, S.A., (1982) *The Pope As Philosopher, Psychiatrist And Healer*, The Sower, London, Summer.

Ward, S.A., (1985) *Stressful Pregnancies and Traumatic Births Resulting In Possible Behaviour, Emotional And Learning Difficulties*. Unpublished Masters Thesis. Nottingham University, UK.

Ward, S.A., (1999) *Birth Trauma in Infants and Children*. Journal of Prenatal and Perinatal Psychology and Health. Volume 13 (3-4) p 201 – 212. USA

Ward, S.A., (2004) *Suicide and Pre and Perinatal Psychotherapy Journal of Pre and Perinatal Psychology and Health*. Volume 19 (2) 2004 p 89 – 105.

Ward, S.A., (2011) *Global Fractal Waves*. Inside Out:Journal of the Association Of Humanistic and Integrative Psychotherapy Summer Issue Number 64 IAHIP Dun Laoghaire, County Dublin, Ireland. (see www.iahip.org)

Ward, S.(2014). *Fractals From The Womb: A Journey Through pre- and Perinatal Psychotherapy*. Author: Shirley Ward. Re-published 2019 by Twin Flame Productions, Oregon (https://twinflameproductions.us) as *Healing Birth Healing Earth*.

Wasdell, D., (1998) *The First Trimester*, Urchin, London.

White, R., (1993) *Working With Your Chakras*, Piatkus.

Whitfield, C., (1987) *Healing the Child Within*. Health Communications. Deerfield Beach: USA
Whitfield, C., (1993) *Boundaries and Relationships*. Health Communications. Deerfield Beach: USA
Whitfield, G.V., (2007) *The Prenatal Psychology of Frank Lake And The Origins of Sin and Human Dysfunction*. Emeth Press. Lexington, USA.
Wilber, K., (1979) *Are The Chakras Real?* In White, J. (Ed.), Kundlini, Evolution and Enlightenment. Doubleday/Anchor.
Wilber, K., (1980) *The Atman Project: A Transpersonal View of Human Development*. A Quest Book.
Winnicott, D., (1965) E*go Distortion in Terms of True and False Self in The Maturational Processes and the Facilitating Environment.*
Woodman, M., & Dickson, E. (1997) *Dancing in the Flames*. Gill and Macmillan.
Woodward, J., (1998) *The Lone Twin: Understanding Twin Bereavement and Loss*. Free Association Books.

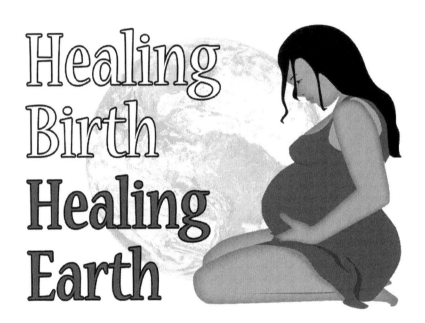

FURTHER INFORMATION

Amethyst
www.holistic.ie/amethyst

Association for Prenatal and Perinatal Psychology and Health
www.birthpsychology.com

Bridge Pastoral Foundation (formerly the Clinical Theology Association)
admin@bridgepastoral.org.uk

Jean Houston
www.jeanhouston.org

Shirley Ward
Web: shirleyward.org **Email:** shirley@shirleyward.org

More To Explore

One important positive fractal that has happened since this conversation took place in September 2018, is that I have booked a little 7-inch plot for my ashes to be interred in Glenstal Benedictines Abbey new Garden Cemetery when I decide to leave! I was not conscious of the link, having been conceived by my parents in the family home in the shadow of the medieval Benedictine Monastery of Peterborough Cathedral, the fractal of sacredness, peace and tranquillity has permeated my life amidst the turmoil of war and trauma. What mysteries life and death have in store for us!

A life learning lesson for me is:
"To help one person heal their birth is to help to save the earth".

This is Book One in the **Healing Birth to Save the Earth** series.
The second book in the series is **Birth, Earth and Our Future**.
The third book in the series is **Global Healing**.

Details of all books/workshops/courses from https://shirleyward.org

Thank you! Shirley Ward

Printed in Great Britain
by Amazon